ΙΠΠΟΚΡΑΤΟΥΣ
ΟΡΚΟΣ

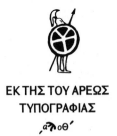

ΕΚ ΤΗΣ ΤΟΥ ΑΡΕΩΣ
ΤΥΠΟΓΡΑΦΙΑΣ
,αϡοθ´

HIPPOCRATES,
THE OATH.

OR

THE HIPPOCRATIC OATH

INTRODUCTION
GREEK TEXT WITH FACING
ENGLISH TRANSLATION, COMMENTARY
AND INTERPRETATION
BY
LUDWIG EDELSTEIN
WITH
AN APPENDIX ON **THE HIPPOCRATIC
PATIENT AND HIS PHYSICIAN** BY
HERBERT NEWELL COUCH

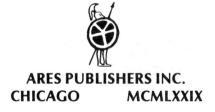

ARES PUBLISHERS INC.
CHICAGO   MCMLXXIX

Exact Reprint of the Edition
Baltimore 1943
ARES PUBLISHERS, INC.
Chicago, Ill.
ISBN 0-89005-272-7

CONTENTS

INTRODUCTION

That for centuries the so-called Hippocratic Oath was the exemplar of medical etiquette and as such determined the professional attitude of generations of physicians, no one will doubt. Yet when it is asked what historical forces were instrumental in the formulation of this document, no answer can be given that is generally agreed upon. Uncertainty still prevails concerning the time when the Oath was composed and concerning the purpose for which it was intended. The dates proposed in modern debate vary from the 6th century B. C. to the 1st century A. D. As for the original intent of the manifesto, it is maintained that the Oath was administered in family guilds of physicians; or that it formed the statute of societies of artisans which perhaps were organized in secret; or that it was an ideal program designed without regard for any particular time or place.

In my opinion it is not necessary to resign oneself to leaving the issue undecided. If some data provided by the text itself are evaluated in their true import and are combined with others the proper meaning of which has previously been established, it seems possible to determine the origin of the Hippocratic Oath with a fair degree of certainty. At any rate, it is with this aim in mind that I propose to re-examine the document.

In so doing I shall scrutinize the Hippocratic text sentence by sentence—the treatise is short enough to allow completeness of interpretation—for it is only in this way that the adequacy or inadequacy of the thesis to be offered can be tested. Moreover, I shall give in full the testimony of ancient authors on which I depend in my inquiry. The material used is scattered and in some cases difficult of access, and it should be at hand if the cogency of the argument is to be judged. Such a method of investigation necessarily results in a certain copiousness, but this hardly needs justification in view of the importance of the Hippocratic Oath, both for the history of medicine and of ethics.

TEXT AND TRANSLATION *

* Text and Apparatus Criticus are taken from *Hippocratis Opera*, ed. I. L. Heiberg, *Corpus Medicorum Graecorum* I, 1, 1927, pp. 4-5.

ΟΡΚΟΣ

Ὀμνύω Ἀπόλλωνα ἰητρὸν καὶ Ἀσκληπιὸν καὶ Ὑγείαν καὶ Πανάκειαν
καὶ θεοὺς πάντας τε καὶ πάσας ἴστορας ποιεύμενος ἐπιτελέα ποιήσειν κατὰ
δύναμιν καὶ κρίσιν ἐμὴν ὅρκον τόνδε καὶ ξυγγραφὴν τήνδε·

5 ἡγήσασθαί τε τὸν διδάξαντά με τὴν τέχνην ταύτην ἴσα γενέτῃσιν
ἐμοῖσιν καὶ βίου κοινώσασθαι καὶ χρεῶν χρηίζοντι μετάδοσιν ποιήσασθαι
καὶ γένος τὸ ἐξ αὐτοῦ ἀδελφεοῖς ἴσον ἐπικρινέειν ἄρρεσι καὶ διδάξειν τὴν
τέχνην ταύτην, ἢν χρηίζωσι μανθάνειν, ἄνευ μισθοῦ καὶ ξυγγραφῆς, παραγγελίης τε καὶ ἀκροήσιος καὶ τῆς λοιπῆς ἁπάσης μαθήσιος μετάδοσιν
10 ποιήσασθαι υἱοῖσί τε ἐμοῖσι καὶ τοῖσι τοῦ ἐμὲ διδάξαντος καὶ μαθηταῖσι
συγγεγραμμένοις τε καὶ ὡρκισμένοις νόμῳ ἰητρικῷ, ἄλλῳ δὲ οὐδενί.

διαιτήμασί τε χρήσομαι ἐπ᾽ ὠφελείῃ καμνόντων κατὰ δύναμιν καὶ κρίσιν
ἐμήν· ἐπὶ δηλήσει δὲ καὶ ἀδικίῃ εἴρξειν.

οὐ δώσω δὲ οὐδὲ φάρμακον οὐδενὶ αἰτηθεὶς θανάσιμον οὐδὲ ὑφηγήσομαι
15 ξυμβουλίην τοιήνδε· ὁμοίως δὲ οὐδὲ γυναικὶ πεσσὸν φθόριον δώσω. ἁγνῶς
δὲ καὶ ὁσίως διατηρήσω βίον ἐμὸν καὶ τέχνην ἐμήν.

οὐ τεμέω δὲ οὐδὲ μὴν λιθιῶντας, ἐκχωρήσω δὲ ἐργάτῃσιν ἀνδράσιν
πρήξιος τῆσδε.

ἐς οἰκίας δὲ ὁκόσας ἂν ἐσίω, ἐσελεύσομαι ἐπ᾽ ὠφελείῃ καμνόντων ἐκτὸς
20 ἐὼν πάσης ἀδικίης ἑκουσίης καὶ φθορίης τῆς τε ἄλλης καὶ ἀφροδισίων
ἔργων ἐπί τε γυναικείων σωμάτων καὶ ἀνδρείων ἐλευθέρων τε καὶ δούλων.

ἃ δ᾽ ἂν ἐν θεραπείῃ ἢ ἴδω ἢ ἀκούσω ἢ καὶ ἄνευ θεραπηίης κατὰ βίον
ἀνθρώπων, ἃ μὴ χρή ποτε ἐκλαλέεσθαι ἔξω, σιγήσομαι ἄρρητα ἡγεύμενος
εἶναι τὰ τοιαῦτα.

25 ὅρκον μὲν οὖν μοι τόνδε ἐπιτελέα ποιέοντι καὶ μὴ ξυγχέοντι εἴη ἐπαύ-
ρασθαι καὶ βίου καὶ τέχνης δοξαζομένῳ παρὰ πᾶσιν ἀνθρώποις ἐς τὸν
αἰεὶ χρόνον, παραβαίνοντι δὲ καὶ ἐπιορκοῦντι τἀναντία τουτέων.

Titulus: ἱπποκράτους ὅρκος M V R U *Mg.* ᾱ' V   2 ὄμνυμι R U   3 ἅπαντας V τε]
om. V *Supra* ἴστορας *scr.* μάρτυρας U, *m. rec.* R ποίησιν V   4 συγγραφὴν *supra scr.*
ξ V, *supra add.* συμφωνίαν U, *m. rec.* R   5 τε] V, δὲ M R U, μὲν *Littré* ἴσα γενέτῃσιν]
ἴσα καὶ γενέτοισιν R U   6 ἐμοῖσι V R U χρέους V, χρέος? *Diels* χρήξοντι V   7 καὶ
γένος — ποιήσασθαι (10) *om.* V αὐτοῦ] *Ermerins*, ἑωυτέου M R, ὡυτέου U ἀδελφοῖς U
ἀποκρινέειν U, *sed corr.*   8 *Supra* ξυγγραφῆς *scr.* συμφωνίας U, *m. rec.* R   8-9 *Supra*
παραγγελίης *scr.* παρακλῆ *m. rec.* R, παρακλήσεως U   10 τοῖσι] *in Mg. transiens* U
11 *supra* συγγεγραμμένοις *scr.* συμφωνίαν δοῦσι R τε] euan. V ὡρκιζομένοις M, *sed corr.*
13 *Supra* δηλήσει *scr.* βλάβῃ U   14 *supra* ὑφηγήσομαι *scr.* ὑποβαλῶ *m. rec.*, *mg.* ὑπο-
θήσομαι συμβουλεύσω R   15 φθόριον δώσω πεσσόν R U   1⟨ ἐμὸν] τὸν ἐμὸν R U ἐμήν]
τὴν ἐμὴν R U   17 *post* δὲ *lac. statuit Diels* ἀνδράσιν] M, ἀνδράσι V R U   18 πρήξιος
V   19 ἐς] V, εἰς M R U καμνόντων] κα- *in ras.* U   21 ἀνδρείων] V M ², ἀνδρίων M,
ἀνδρώων R U   22 *pr.* ἢ *om.* V θεραπηίης V   23 ἐκκαλέεσθαι U   24 τὰ τοιαῦτα εἶναι V
25 ποιέοντι] -έο- *in ras mai.* U   26 εἰς M R U *In fine:* ὅρκος M V

2

OATH

I swear by Apollo Physician and Asclepius and Hygieia and Panaceia and all the gods and goddesses, making them my witnesses, that I will fulfil according to my ability and judgment this oath and this covenant:

To hold him who has taught me this art as equal to my parents and to live my life in partnership with him, and if he is in need of money to give him a share of mine, and to regard his offspring as equal to my brothers in male lineage and to teach them this art—if they desire to learn it—without fee and covenant; to give a share of precepts and oral instruction and all the other learning to my sons and to the sons of him who has instructed me and to pupils who have signed the covenant and have taken an oath according to the medical law, but to no one else.

I will apply dietetic measures for the benefit of the sick according to my ability and judgment; I will keep them from harm and injustice.

I will neither give a deadly drug to anybody if asked for it, nor will I make a suggestion to this effect. Similarly I will not give to a woman an abortive remedy. In purity and holiness I will guard my life and my art.

I will not use the knife, not even on sufferers from stone, but will withdraw in favor of such men as are engaged in this work.

Whatever houses I may visit, I will come for the benefit of the sick, remaining free of all intentional injustice, of all mischief and in particular of sexual relations with both female and male persons, be they free or slaves.

What I may see or hear in the course of the treatment or even outside of the treatment in regard to the life of men, which on no account one must spread abroad, I will keep to myself holding such things shameful to be spoken about.

If I fulfil this oath and do not violate it, may it be granted to me to enjoy life and art, being honored with fame among all men for all time to come; if I transgress it and swear falsely, may the opposite of all this be my lot.

3

INTERPRETATION

The Hippocratic Oath clearly falls into two parts. The first specifies the duties of the pupil towards his teacher and his teacher's family and the pupil's obligations in transmitting medical knowledge.[1] The second gives a number of rules to be observed in the treatment of diseases, a short summary of medical ethics as it were.[2] Most scholars consider these two sections to be only superficially connected or at least determined by different moral standards.[3] Be this as it may, the two parts certainly diverge in their subject matter, and, for the purpose of analyzing their content, it is advantageous first to discuss them separately and then to ask how they are related to each other. Again for the sake of convenience, I shall deal with the so-called ethical code first, the main question being whether the historical setting in which these rules of conduct were conceived can be ferreted out.

Modern interpreters are wont to see in the ethical provisions of the Oath the expression of certain general principles the recognition of which is demanded by human decency or by the responsibilities inherent in the physician's art. In this sense timeless validity is usually attributed to the moral law here established.[4] At best such an evaluation is qualified by the admission that the Oath represents only the ancient ideal of the physician. Justice is enjoined upon him, it is said, in contrast to charity that motivates the Christian doctor, and in contrast to duty towards the community that determines the doctor of today.[5] Even if such characterizations were correct, it

---

[1] Cf. above, pp. 2, 5-11.   [2] Cf. above, pp. 2, 12-24.

[3] Cf. *e. g.* W. H. S. Jones, *The Doctor's Oath*, 1924, p. 56; K. Deichgräber, Die ärztliche Standesethik des hippokratischen Eides, *Quellen u. Studien z. Geschichte d. Naturwissenschaften u. d. Medizin*, III, 1932, p. 34. Cf. also below, p. 50.

[4] Cf. *e. g.* Jones, *op. cit.*, p. 46: " Custom and convenience, to say nothing of the human conscience, would sooner or later lay down most of the rules of conduct comprised in *Oath* . . ."; cf. also p. 50: ". . . the appeal to his (*sc.* the Greek doctor's) better feelings." Cf. also O. Körner, *Der Eid des Hippokrates*, 1921, p. 20: " Alle diese Gelöbnisse dienen allein dem Wohle der Kranken und keinen Sonderinteressen der Ärzte. Erschöpfend umfassen sie in grossen Zügen, was der Arzt dem Kranken schuldet."

[5] Cf. Deichgräber, *op. cit.*, pp. 38 ff.; esp. pp. 41 ff. (" Die Idee des δίκαιος ἰατρός ist in den Bestimmungen des Eides Gestalt geworden, wenn man so will, die Idee des apollinischen Arztes " [p. 42]).

4

would not be superfluous to ask when and where this supposedly general attitude towards medicine and its tasks was codified. Besides, it is only by uncovering the specific ethical agents which brought about this formulation that the origin of the Oath can be ascertained.

Unfortunately, most of the statements contained in the document are worded in rather general terms; they are vague in their commending of justice, of purity and holiness, concepts which in themselves do not imply any distinct meaning but may be understood in various ways. Yet there are two stipulations that have a more definite character and seem to point to the basic beliefs underlying the whole program which is here evolved: the rules concerning the application of poison and of abortive remedies. Their interpretation should therefore provide a clue for a historical identification of the views embodied in the Oath of Hippocrates.

I

THE ETHICAL CODE

A

Rules concerning Poison and Abortion

"I will neither give a deadly drug to anybody if asked for it, nor will I make a suggestion to this effect. Similarly I will not give to a woman an abortive remedy. In purity and holiness I will guard my life and my art " — such is the vow made.[1] It concerns the physician not so much in his capacity as the healer of diseases but rather in that of the pharmacist who is in possession of the drugs which he prescribes. Poison is a drug and so is the pessary.[2] The physician agrees not to deliver either one to his patient. The term used in both instances is the same; just as he will not *give* the pessary to a woman who comes to seek his help, he will not *give* poison to anyone who is under his care.[3]

Why regulations concerning cases of abortion are introduced into the document is immediately understandable. Under ancient conditions the physician was often presented with the problem as to whether he should give an abortive remedy.[4] But what about the physician's supplying poison? Did he so frequently have occasion to

[1] Cf. above, pp. 2, 14-16.

[2] E. Littré, *Œuvres complètes d'Hippocrate*, IV, 1844, pp. 622 ff., has shown that this clause presupposes a state of affairs in which the physician was his own apothecary. This he was even in those centuries in which pharmacies existed, cf. *e. g.* Galen, *Opera*, ed. C. G. Kühn, XIV, 1827, pp. 5 ff. For the pessary, a "Stäbchen . . . mit bestimmten φάρμακα bestrichen," cf. Deichgräber, *op. cit.*, n. 10.

[3] As far as I am aware, Littré was the first to suggest another meaning of the sentence in question. He says, *op. cit.*, IV, p. 630, n. 12, in commenting on δώσω— the word I have translated by *give*—: "Les traducteurs rendent δώσω par *propinabo* (*sc.* in the first stipulation) ; mais δώσω, qui, un peu plus bas (*sc.* in the second instance), est joint à πεσσός, et qui là ne peut se rendre par *administrer*, montre que dans les deux cas il s'agit d'une substance malfaisante remise à des tiers. . . ." Littré seems to have believed that no physician could possibly give a pessary to his patient directly. But as C. Daremberg, *Œuvres choisis d'Hippocrate*[2], 1855, p. 9, later pointed out, ancient physicians did do so, and it is in connection with the Hippocratic Oath that it was discussed whether this was right; cf. below, pp. 11 f. Littré's reasoning for his interpretation then is not valid.

[4] For abortion as a general practice in antiquity, cf. below, p. 10.

give poison that it seemed worth while to ordain what he should do in such instances? What exactly is the situation referred to in the Oath?

All modern interpreters assume that the interdiction of the supplying of poisons means that the physician is charged not to assist his patient in a suicide which he might contemplate. Some interpreters claim that here the physician is also, or even primarily, asked to refrain from any criminal attempt on his patient's life. Cases of poisoning, they say, were very frequent in antiquity; the law, though of course it threatened punishment for murder, was of little avail because the lack of proper scientific methods made it impossible to ascertain whether poison had been administered or not. As a means of strengthening civil jurisdiction, therefore, a clause was introduced into the ancient medical code which today would be entirely out of place.[5] I shall not argue that the Greeks could hardly have been aware of that inability to cope with the situation under discussion which resulted from their ignorance of *post-mortem* examinations and modern chemistry. As a matter of fact they were convinced that they were quite capable of detecting such a crime as poisoning and the criminal who had perpetrated it.[6] More important, if the prohibition were instigated by the wish of society to defend itself against a pernicious assault, then the rules given would be concerned not with the doctor's attitude towards his patient but towards a third party. For the patient himself certainly would not ask his doctor for the poison with which he is to be murdered, and yet the physician vows not to give poison when asked to do so. There is no evidence, however, that the Oath refers to anybody except patient and physi-

---

[5] Cf. Littré, *op. cit.*, IV, pp. 622 ff.; Deichgräber, *op. cit.*, p. 36 (Deichgräber apparently accepts Littré's conception of the motive as well as his explanation). It is often overlooked that Littré admits the probability that suicide is also referred to here, but cf. *op. cit.*, IV, p. 630, n. 12. Jones, *op. cit.*, p. 50, is the only one who seems to exclude the latter possibility.

[6] Cf. L. Lewin, *Die Gifte in der Weltgeschichte,* 1920, pp. 37 ff., where ancient methods of determining cases of poisoning are discussed. Besides, torture of those who were suspected was an excellent substitute for scientific inquiry into the case, cf. Apuleius, *Metamorphoses,* X, 10. Note moreover the harshness of Plato, *Laws,* XI, 932 e ff., in dealing with such a crime, especially when committed by a doctor. As understood by most interpreters the stipulation of the *Oath* would be a useless duplication of the existing laws.

8 THE HIPPOCRATIC OATH

cian.[7] The words in question, then, can mean only that the doctor promises not to supply his patient with poison if asked by him to do so nor to suggest that he take it. It is the prevention of suicide, not of murder, that is here implied.[8]

But was suicide an instance to be reckoned with in medical practice? Could the doctor ever advise such an act to his patient? In antiquity this was indeed the case. If the sick felt that their pains had become intolerable, if no help could be expected, they often put an end to their own lives. This fact is repeatedly attested and not only in general terms; even the diseases are specified which in the opinion of the ancients gave justification for a voluntary death.[9]

[7] Cf. above, p. 6, n. 3. Littré is well aware of the fact that his interpretation necessitates a reference to a third person (op. cit., IV, p. 623-24); cf. also J. E. Pétrequin, Chirurgie d'Hippocrate, I, 1877, p. 185. Deichgräber, loc. cit., and Jones, loc. cit., do not discuss at all the problem as to whom this stipulation refers. Nor have the modern interpreters pondered over the difficulty that on their assumption, according to which the clause concerns suicide as well as murder, the statement is logically incoherent; for in one instance the patient would be referred to, in the other somebody outside the physician's practice.

[8] Cf. Daremberg, op. cit., p. 9: ". . . l'ensemble de la phrase ne me laisse aucun doute sur cette interprétation." The old Latin and Arabic translations of the Oath reproduced by Jones, op. cit., p. 35; p. 31, seem to presuppose the same meaning. (It is hardly necessary to add that in regard to the issue at stake one cannot possibly draw any conclusion from an undated pharmacological poem whose dependence on the Hippocratic Oath cannot be proved, as Deichgräber himself admits, op. cit., p. 36, n. 33.) Most important: Scribonius Largus urges that the physician should not murder anyone, not even his enemy (p. 2, l. 19 ff. Helmreich). In confirmation of such a postulate he quotes the Hippocratic Oath in the following way: "Hippocrates, conditor nostrae professionis, initia disciplinae ab iureiurando tradidit, in quo sanctum est, ne praegnati quidem medicamentum, quo conceptum excutitur, aut detur aut demonstretur a quoquam medico, longe praeformans animos discentium ad humanitatem. qui enim nefas existimaverit spem dubiam hominis laedere, quanto scelestius perfecto iam nocere iudicabit" (p. 2, l. 27–p. 3, l. 2)? It would be meaningless for Scribonius to argue in such a complicated and indirect manner, if the Oath outlined a criminal assault expressis verbis.

[9] Cf. e.g. Aristotle, E.E., 1229 b 39: ". . . οὔτ' εἰ φεύγοντες τὸ πονεῖν, ὅπερ πολλοὶ ποιοῦσιν, οὐδὲ τῶν τοιούτων οὐδεὶς ἀνδρεῖος, καθάπερ καὶ 'Αγάθων φησί· 'φαῦλοι βροτῶν γὰρ τοῦ πονεῖν ἡσσώμενοι/θανεῖν ἐρῶσιν.' ὥσπερ καὶ τὸν Χείρωνα μυθολογοῦσιν οἱ ποιηταὶ διὰ τὴν ἀπὸ τοῦ ἕλκους ὀδύνην εὔξασθαι ἀποθανεῖν ἀθάνατον ὄντα. The reference to Chiron and his disease makes it certain that the term τὸ πονεῖν means "to suffer bodily pains," cf. also below pp. 14 f. Cf. also Pliny, Nat. Hist., XX, 199: "Sic scimus interemptum P. Licini Caecinae praetorii viri patrem in Hispania Bavili, cum valetudo inpetibilis odium vitae fecisset; item plerosque alios." For the diseases in question cf. Pliny, Nat. Hist., XXV, 23: "Qui (sc. morbi) gravis-

Moreover, the taking of poison was the most usual means of committing suicide, and the patient was likely to demand the poison from his physician who was in possession of deadly drugs and knew those which brought about an easy and painless end.[10] On the other hand, such a resolution naturally was not taken without due deliberation, except perhaps in a few cases of great distress or mental strain. The sick wished to be sure that further treatment would be of no avail, and to render this verdict was the physician's task. The patient, therefore, consulted with him, or urged his friends to speak to the doctor. If the latter, in such a consultation, confirmed the seriousness or hopelessness of the case, he suggested directly or indirectly that the patient commit suicide.[11]

Of course, I do not mean to claim that everybody whose illness had become desperate thought of ending his own life. Even if human aid was no longer effectual, recourse to the gods was still possible, and men did seek succor in the sanctuaries; even if the pain was

simi ex his sint, discernere stultitiae prope videri possit, cum suus cuique ac praesens quisque atrocissimus videatur. et de hoc tamen iudicavere aevi experimenta, asperrimi cruciatus esse calculorum a stillicidio vesicae, proximum stomachi, tertium eorum, quae in capite doleant, non ob alios fere morte conscita."

[10] For poison commonly used in suicide, cf. Lewin, *op. cit.*, p. 139; p. 65. For instances where poison is demanded from the physician, cf. *e. g. Scriptores Historiae Augustae, Vita Hadriani*, 24, 13; Tacitus, *Annals*, XV, 64; Apuleius, *Metamorphoses*, X, 9. Even Theophrastus, *Hist. Plant.*, IX, 16, 8, speaks of men who invented especially efficacious and painless poisons for suicide; since he says that these people were also versed in all other branches of medicine it is not necessary to understand with Littré, *op. cit.*, IV, p. 622, that they were merely vendors of drugs. They may just as well have been physicians.

[11] Cf. Pliny, *Epistulae*, I, xxii, 7 ff.: "Mirareris, si interesses, qua patientia hanc ipsam valitudinem toleret, ut dolori resistat, ut sitim differat, ut incredibilem febrium ardorem inmotus opertusque transmittat. nuper me paucosque mecum quos maxime diligit advocavit rogavitque ut medicos consuleremus de summa valitudinis, ut, si esset insuperabilis, sponte exiret e vita, si tantum difficilis et longa, resisteret maneretque: dandum enim precibus uxoris, dandum filiae lacrimis, dandum etiam nobis amicis ne spes nostras, si modo non essent inanes, voluntaria morte desereret. id ego arduum in primis et praecipua laude dignum puto. nam impetu quodam et instinctu procurrere ad mortem commune cum multis, deliberare vero et causas eius expendere, utque suaserit ratio, vitae mortisque consilium vel suscipere vel ponere ingentis est animi. et medici quidem secunda nobis pollicentur." This passage, the importance of which is rightly stressed by A. W. Mair, *Encyclopaedia of Religion and Ethics, s. v.* suicide, XII, pp. 31-32, certainly is tinged with Stoic feeling. But there is no reason to doubt that earlier generations were as cautious and responsible in making their decisions as were the Romans.

excruciating and relief was to be had neither from human nor from divine physicians, men could, and did go on living in spite of all their suffering.[12] ᵗYet the fact remains that throughout antiquity many people preferred voluntary death to endless agony. This form of " euthanasia " was an everyday reality.[13] |Consequently it is quite understandable that the Oath deals withᶦ the attitude which the physician should take in regard to the possible suicide of his patient. From a practical point of view it was no less important to tell the ancient doctor what to do when faced with such a situation than it was to advise him about cases of abortion.[14]

The relevance of the " pharmacological rules " for a medical oath having been established, one may now ask why the Oath forbids the physician to assist in suicide or in abortion. |Apparently these prohibitions did not echo the general feeling of the public. Suicide was not censured in antiquity.[15] Abortion wa's practiced in Greek times no less than in the Roman era, and it was resorted to without scruple. Small wonder! In a world in which it was held justifiable to expose children immediately after birth, it would hardly seem objectionable to destroy the embryo.[16] Why then should the physician not give a helping hand to those of his patients who wanted to end their own lives or to those who did not wish to have offspring?

[12] For the seeking of religious help in hopeless cases, cf. L. Edelstein, Greek Medicine in its Relation to Religion and Magic, *Bulletin of the History of Medicine,* V, 1937, pp. 238 ff. For instances of rejection of suicide cf. below p. 14.

[13] Strangely enough none of the interpreters of the *Oath* has pointed to this fact. Deichgräber, the only one to mention the problem of euthanasia, *op. cit.,* p. 36, even denies that it had any importance for the ancients. The writers on suicide, on the other hand, though they refer to voluntary death on account of illness, do not mention the *Oath,* cf. *e. g.* R. Hirzel, Der Selbstmord, *Archiv f. Religionswissenschaft,* XI, 1908, pp. 75 ff.; 243 ff.; 417 ff.; *E. R. E., s. v.* suicide, XII, pp. 26 b ff.

[14] In my opinion it is the neglect of the question of euthanasia that gave currency to the belief that in the *Oath* not only suicide but also manslaughter are forbidden (cf. Deichgräber, *op. cit.,* p. 36: " *Da* das Euthanasieproblem, an das der moderne Mensch denken könnte, in der Antike unbekannt ist, *kann* es sich hier *nur* um den Giftmord und als einen besonderen Fall, den durch Gift herbeigeführten Selbstmord sowie um die Beihilfe zu beidem handeln." [Italics mine.]).

[15] Cf. above, pp. 8 ff., and below, pp. 13 ff.

[16] Cf. in general A. E. Crawley, *E. R. E., s. v.* foeticide, VI, pp. 54 b ff. For the parental power over children of which exposure after birth and destruction of the embryo are the consequences, cf. Wilamowitz, *Staat u. Gesellschaft der Griechen, Die Kultur der Gegenwart,* II, IV, 1², 1923, p. 36.

For a moment one might harbor the idea that the interdiction of poison and of abortive remedies was simply the outgrowth of medical ethics. After all, medicine is the art of healing, of preserving life. Should the physician assist in bringing about death?[17] I do not propose to discuss this issue in general terms. It suffices here to state that in antiquity many physicians actually gave their patients the poison for which they were asked. Apparently *qua* physicians they felt no compunction about doing so.[18] Although in later centuries some refused to participate in an attempt on men's lives, because, as they said, it was unfitting for their sect "to be responsible for anyone's death or destruction,"[19] it is not reported that they ever employed the same reasoning in cases of self-murder.[20] As for abortions, many physicians prescribed and gave abortive remedies. Medical writings of all periods mention the means for the destruction of the embryo and the occasions where they are to be employed.[21]

[17] It is permissible to say that this is the most commonly accepted explanation of the rules, cf. *e. g.* Körner, *op. cit.*, p. 12: "Seine· (*sc.* the physician's) höchste Aufgabe ist Heilen, und sein schlimmstes Verbrechen wäre also Töten oder Vorschubleisten zu Mord, Selbstmord und Kindesabtreibung."

[18] Cf. *e. g.* Tacitus, *Annals*, XV, 64; cf. also Apuleius, *Metamorphoses*, X, 9, where the physician is approached for poison by a slave, and since he becomes suspicious, gives him a harmless drug only. But he is not astonished about the demand made, nor does he refuse it on general grounds. This can easily be explained, for those suffering from incurable diseases were doomed to die anyhow; the only issue was, whether they should be condemned to an unnecessarily protracted suffering. Moreover, death seemed desirable to the sick, and even the Hippocratic maxim "to help, or at least not to do harm" (*Epidemiae*, I, 11, *Hippocratis Opera*, ed. H. Kuehlewein, I, 1894, p. 190) could not restrain the physician when he was face to face with those who believed that they would be helped rather than harmed by annihilation.

[19] Cf. Apuleius, *Metamorphoses*, X, 11; note that these are the words of the same physician who before (X, 9, cf. preceding note) did not reject the giving of poison to a suicide.

[20] This assertion, of course, is not refuted by the fact that in Oxyrhynchus Papyrus 437 (III, 77, 3rd century A. D.) the giving of poison is rejected as incompatible with the art by a quotation from the *Oath*; cf. Deichgräber, *op. cit.*, n. 42. Through this document the interdiction of poison became part of medical ethics; that does not mean, however, that originally it was the outgrowth of medical considerations.

[21] Cf. R. Hähnel, Der künstliche Abortus im Altertum, *Archiv f. Geschichte d. Medizin*, XXIX, 1937, pp. 224 ff. J. Ilberg, Zur gynäkologischen Ethik der Griechen, *Archiv f. Religionswissenschaft*, XIII, 1910, pp. 12 ff., holds that the Greek physicians did not apply abortive remedies; but this thesis is untenable in

In later centuries some physicians rejected abortion under all circumstances; they supported their decision with a reference to the prohibition in the Hippocratic Oath and added that it was the duty of the doctor to preserve the products of nature. Soranus, the greatest of the ancient gynaecologists, had little patience with these colleagues of his. In agreement with many other physicians he contended that it was necessary to think of the life of the mother first, and he resorted to abortion whenever it seemed necessary, much as he deprecated it if performed for no other reason than the wish to preserve beauty or to hide the consequences of adultery.[22] In short, the strict attitude upheld by the Oath was not uncontested even from the medical point of view. In antiquity it was not generally considered a violation of medical ethics to do what the Oath forbade. An ancient doctor who accepted the rules laid down by "Hippocrates" was by no means in agreement with the opinion of all his fellow physicians; on the contrary, he adhered to a dogma which was much stricter than that embraced by many, if not by most of his colleagues. Simple reflection on the duties of the physician, on the task of medicine alone, under these circumstances, can hardly have led to the formulation and adoption of the "pharmacological stipulations."

In my opinion, the Oath itself points to other, more fundamental considerations that must have been instrumental in outlining the prohibitions under discussion. For the physician, when forswearing the use of poison and of abortive remedies, adds: "In purity and in holiness I will guard my life and my art."[23] It might be possible to construe purity as a quality insisted upon by the craftsman who is conscious of the obligations of his art. The demand for holiness,

view of the facts now conveniently surveyed by R. Hähnel, *loc. cit.*; cf. also Deichgräber, *op. cit.*, n. 37; P. Diepgen, *Die Frauenheilkunde der Alten Welt*, 1937, p. 301.

[22] Cf. Soranus, ed. J. Ilberg, *C.M.G.*, IV, 1927, p. 45, 8 ff. Incidentally the passage in Soranus proves that the rejection of abortion as advocated in the *Oath* is laid down without qualification (contrary to the assumption made by F. J. Dölger, *Antike u. Christentum*, IV, 1934, p. 8).

[23] Cf. above, pp. 2, 15-16. It is interesting to note that Körner who sees in these stipulations the expression of medical ethics (cf. above p. 4, n. 4) translates ἀγνῶς δὲ καὶ ὁσίως with "ohne Fehl und unbescholten" (*op. cit.*, p. 5), a translation which in no way does justice to the meaning of the words. All other interpreters in their rendering rightly reflect the notions of holiness and purity.

however, can hardly be understood as resulting from practical thinking or technical responsibility. Holiness belongs to another realm of
values and is indicative of standards of a different, a more elevated
character.

Yet certainly not such purity and holiness are meant as might
accrue to men from obedience to civil law or common religion.
Ancient jurisdiction did not discriminate against suicide; it did not
attach any disgrace to it, provided that there was sufficient reason for
such an act. And self-murder as a relief from illness was regarded
as justifiable, so much so that in some states it was an institution
duly legalized by the authorities.[24] Nor did Greek or Roman law
protect the unborn child. If, in certain cities, abortion was prose-
cuted, it was because the father's right to his offspring had been
violated by the mother's action.[25] Ancient religion did not proscribe
suicide. It did not know of any eternal punishment for those who
voluntarily ended their lives.[26] Likewise it remained indifferent to

[24] Cf. Hirzel, op. cit., pp. 264 ff.; E. R. E., loc. cit. The special regulations for
the burial of a suicide in Athens (Aristotle, N. E., 1138 a 9 ff.) have been rightly
explained by Hirzel, ibid., p. 264; 271, as directed against those who committed
suicide when still able to bear arms; the same is true of Rome (ibid., p. 266).
This fact has been overlooked by Deichgräber, op. cit., p. 36, n. 35. Note moreover
that not even these people were deprived of burial. For city regulations concerning
the delivery of poisons to suicides, cf. E. R. E., loc. cit., pp. 28 ff. Temporary
legislation against suicide (cf. Hirzel, ibid., p. 275) indicative of the frequency of
such occurrences was never directed against suicide on account of illness. Thebes
was the only city where, according to late evidence, suicide was forbidden (cf.
Hirzel, ibid., p. 268); for the explanation of this fact, cf. below, p. 18, n. 44.

[25] For lawsuits based on the father's claim to his children, cf. e. g. Lysias, Fr.
X, p. 333 [Thalheim], and Cicero, Pro Cluentio, XI, 32 (for more material,
especially for the Roman centuries, cf. Dölger, op. cit., pp. 37 ff.). Even Dölger,
ibid., p. 13, admits that in these cases the wish to protect the life of the embryo is
not involved, though he is inclined to believe that the Greeks at least knew of laws
against abortion. But the so-called laws of Solon and Lycurgus, quoted only in a
Ps. Galenic book of unknown date and origin (An animal sit id quod in utero est
XIX, p. 179 K.; cf. K. Kalbfleisch, Abh. Berl. Akad., 1895, p. 11, n. 1), to which
Dölger refers, ibid., pp. 10 ff. (cf. also W. Aly, R. E., III A, p. 963), cannot prove
this thesis. They are late inventions, determined by the thought of the Christian
era. Dölger himself, ibid., p. 14, admits such a falsification in the case of Musonius,
Fr. XVa, p. 77H, the only other passage which in general terms speaks of laws
against abortion.

[26] This has been shown conclusively by Hirzel, op. cit., pp. 76 ff.; p. 276; on
later changes under the influence of Jewish-Christian ideas, cf. ibid., p. 277, and
below, p. 17, n. 40. In E. R. E., XII, pp. 30 b ff., after an elaborate proof that

foeticide. Its tenets did not include the dogma of an immortal soul for which men must render account to their creator.[27] Law and religion then left the physician free to do whatever seemed best to him.

From all these considerations it follows that a specific philosophical conviction must have dictated the rules laid down in the Oath. Is it possible to determine this particular philosophy? To take the problem of suicide first: Platonists, Cynics and Stoics can be eliminated at once. They held suicide permissible for the diseased. Some of these philosophers even extolled such an act as the greatest triumph of men over fate.[28] Aristotle, on the other hand, claimed that it was cowardly to give in to bodily pain, and Epicurus admonished men not to be subdued by illness.[29] But does that mean that the Oath is determined by Aristotelian or Epicurean ideas? I shall not insist that it is hard to imagine a physician resisting the adjurations of his patients if he has nothing but Aristotle's or Epicurus' exhortations to courage to quote to them and to himself. It is more important to stress the fact that the Aristotelian and Epicurean opposition to suicide did not involve moral censure. If men decided to take their lives, they were within their rights as sovereign masters of themselves. The Aristotelian and Epicurean schools condoned suicide. Later on the Aristotelians even gave up their leader's teaching, and under the onslaught of the Stoic attack withdrew their disapproval

according to the evidence available suicide was not stigmatized by ancient religious dogma, it is nevertheless assumed that popular religious feeling opposed it. This is due to a non-permissible identification of popular religion with the tenets of one particular sect (the Orphics), cf. below p. 15, n. 33.

[27] Cf. Dölger, *op. cit.*, pp. 15 ff. Here again as in the case of laws against abortion the first indication of its rejection on religious grounds is found in the 1st century A. D. Cf. O. Weinreich, Stiftung u. Kultsatzungen eines Privatheiligtums in Philadelphia in Lydien, *S. B. Heidelb.*, 1919.

[28] For Plato, cf. *Laws*, IX, 873c, and Hirzel, *op. cit.*, p. 279, n. 1; for the Cynics, cf. Hirzel, *ibid.*, pp. 279-80; for the Stoics, cf. especially *Stoicorum Veterum Fragmenta*, ed. H. v. Arnim, III, 1923, pp. 187 ff., and in general E. Benz, Das Todesproblem in der stoischen Philosophie, *Tübinger Beiträge z. Altertumswissenschaft*, VII, 1929, pp. 54 ff. The Cyrenaics too permitted suicide, cf. Hirzel, *op. cit.*, p. 422.

[29] For Aristotle, cf. *N. E.*, 1116 a 12 ff.; for Epicurus, cf. *Fr.* 138 [Usener]. It is debatable whether Epicurus opposed suicide at all, cf. Diogenes Laertius, X, 119, and A. Kochalsky, *Das Leben u. die Lehre des Epikur*, 1914, n. 111; in general Hirzel, *op. cit.*, p. 422; p. 282.

of self-murder.³⁰ At any rate, Aristotelianism and Epicureanism do not explain a rejection of suicide which apparently is based on a moral creed and a belief in the divine.

Pythagoreanism, then, remains the only philosophical dogma that can possibly account for the attitude advocated in the Hippocratic Oath. For indeed among all Greek thinkers the Pythagoreans alone outlawed suicide and did so without qualification. The Platonic Socrates can adduce no other witness than the Pythagorean Philolaus for the view that men, whatever their fate, are not allowed to take their own lives. And even in later centuries the Pythagorean school is the only one represented as absolutely opposed to suicide.³¹ Moreover, for the Pythagorean, suicide was a sin against god who had allocated to man his position in life as a post to be held and to be defended. Punishment threatened those who did not obey the divine command to live; it was considered neither lawful nor holy to seek release, "to bestow this blessing upon oneself." ³² Any physician who accepts such a dogma naturally must abstain from assisting in suicide or even from suggesting it. Otherwise he would be guilty of a crime, he no less than his patient, and in this moral and religious conviction the doctor can well find the courage to remain deaf to his patient's insistence, to his sufferings, and even to the clamor of the world which disagrees almost unanimously with the stand taken by him. It seems safe to state this much: the fact that in the Hippocratic Oath the physician is enjoined to refrain from aiding or advising suicide points to an influence of Pythagorean doctrines.³³

³⁰ Cf. in general Hirzel, op. cit., p. 422. For the later Aristotelians, cf. R. Walzer, Magna Moralia und aristotelische Ethik, Neue Philologische Untersuchungen, VII, 1929, p. 192. ·

³¹ Cf. Phaedo, 61 d ff., and Hirzel, op. cit., p. 278, who is right in saying that this concept is so emphatically formulated because it is expressed here for the first time. Note that the stipulation is laid down even for those οἷς βέλτιον τεθνάναι ἢ ζῆν (62a). For later Pythagoreans, cf. Athenaeus, IV, 157 C (Euxitheus).

³² Cf. Phaedo, 61 d: τὸ μὴ θεμιτὸν εἶναι ἑαυτὸν βιάζεσθαι . . . 62 a: μὴ ὅσιον αὐτοὺς ἑαυτοὺς εὖ ποιεῖν . . . 62 b: ὁ μὲν οὖν ἐν ἀπορρήτοις λεγόμενος περὶ αὐτῶν λόγος, ὡς ἔν τινι φρουρᾷ ἐσμεν οἱ ἄνθρωποι καὶ οὐ δεῖ δὴ ἑαυτὸν ἐκ ταύτης λύειν οὐδ' ἀποδιδράσκειν . . .

³³ I say Pythagorean doctrines. How far this dogma is influenced by Orphism or even dependent upon it, is not for me to decide. J. Burnet, E. R. E., s. v. Pythagoras and Pythagoreanism, X, 526 a-b, holds that Philolaus' view as represented by Plato is different from Orphic beliefs and characterizes as Pythagorean

In my opinion the same can be asserted of the rule forbidding abortion and rejecting it without qualification. Most of the Greek philosophers even commended abortion. For Plato, foeticide is one of the regular institutions of the ideal state. Whenever the parents are beyond that age which he thinks best for the begetting of children, the embryo should be destroyed.[34] Aristotle reckons abortion the best procedure to keep the population within the limits which he considers essential for a well-ordered community.[35]

To be sure, one limitation apparently is recognized by ancient philosophers. Aristotle advocates that abortion should be performed before the foetus has attained animal life; after that time he no longer considers abortion compatible with holiness.[36] But such a restriction is based on the biological notion that the embryo from a certain time on partakes in animal life. Other philosophers and scientists, in fact most of them, including the Platonists and the Stoics, denied that such was the case. Animation, they thought, began at the moment of birth. Therefore, in their opinion, abortion must have been permissible throughout pregnancy.[37]

It was different with the Pythagoreans. They held that the embryo was an animate being from the moment of conception. That they did so is expressly attested by a writer of the 3rd century A. D.[38]

the "higher side" of this teaching, that is, its moral implications. But cf. also I. M. Linforth, *The Arts of Orpheus*, 1941, esp. pp. 168 ff. At any rate, one cannot claim on the basis of the words ἐν ἀπορρήτοις which Plato uses that the rejection of suicide is Orphic rather than Pythagorean (contrary to S. Reinach, Ἄωροι βιαιοθάνατοι, *Archiv f. Religionswissenschaft*, IX, 1906, p. 318). For the present purpose the expression "Pythagorean doctrines" seems justified by the fact that the teaching under discussion is directly ascribed to the Pythagoreans by Plato and other writers; cf. below, pp. 18 f.

[34] Cf. *Republic*, V, 461 c; *Laws*, V, 740 d, and for the interpretation of the latter passage, Diepgen, *op. cit.*, p. 297.

[35] Cf. Aristotle, *Politics*, VII, 1335 b 20 ff.

[36] Cf. Aristotle, *Politics*, VII, 1335 b 25: τὸ γὰρ ὅσιον καὶ τὸ μὴ διωρισμένον τῇ αἰσθήσει καὶ τῷ ζῆν ἔσται. Cf. also Dölger, *op. cit.*, pp. 7 ff.

[37] Cf. *Stoicorum Veterum Fragmenta*, II, p. 213 [Arnim], and also Herophilus (H. Diels, *Doxographi Graeci*, 1929, V, 15, p. 426). Concerning the Platonists and Neo-Platonists who denied animation of the embryo because the soul enters the body from without, cf. Kalbfleisch, *op. cit.*, pp. 5 ff.

[38] Cf. Ps. Galen, Πρὸς Γαῦρον περὶ τοῦ πῶς ἐμψυχοῦται τὰ ἔμβρυα, p. 34, 20 [Kalbfleisch]: εἰ δὲ δυνάμει ζῷον ὡς τὸ δεδεγμένον τὴν ἕξιν ἢ μᾶλλον ζῷον ἐνεργείᾳ ἦν τὸ ἔμβρυον, δύσκολον μὲν τὸν καιρὸν ἀφορίσαι τῆς εἰσκρίσεως καὶ πολύ γε τὸ ἀπίθανον ἕξει καὶ πλασματῶδες ὁποῖος ἂν εἶναι ἀφορισθῇ, τοῦ μὲν ὅταν καταβληθῇ τὸ σπέρμα τὸν

The same can be concluded from the Pythagorean system of physiology as it was outlined in the Hellenistic period by Alexander Polyhistor: the germ is a clot of brain containing hot vapors within it, and soul and sensation are supposed to originate from this vapor. Similar views were previously accepted by Philolaus in the 4th century B. C.[39] Consequently, for the Pythagoreans, abortion, whenever practiced, meant destruction of a living being. Granted that the righteousness of abortion depends on whether the embryo is animate or not, the Pythagoreans could not but reject abortion unconditionally.[40]

Furthermore, abortion was irreconcilable with their ethical beliefs no less than with their scientific views. In their ascetic rigorism, in their strictness concerning sexual matters and regarding matrimony in particular, they went farther than any other sect. They banned extramarital relations. Even in matrimony coitus was held justifiable only for the purpose of producing offspring.[41] Besides, children

καιρὸν τοῦτον ἀποδιδόντος ὡς ἂν μηδ' οἵου τε ὄντος ἐν τῇ μήτρᾳ γονίμως κρατηθῆναι μήτι γε ψυχῆς ἔξωθεν τῇ εἰσκρίσει ἑαυτῆς τὴν σύμφυσιν ἀπεργασαμένης—κἀνταῦθα πολὺς ὁ Νουμήνιος καὶ οἱ τὰς Πυθαγόρου ὑπονοίας ἐξηγούμενοι . . . The author of the book is Porphyry, cf. Kalbfleisch, ibid.; p. 25.

[39] Cf. Diogenes Laertius, VIII, 28-9. Kalbfleisch, op. cit., p. 80 ad p. 34, 26 (cf. E. Zeller, Die Philosophie d. Griechen, III, 2³, 1881, pp. 89 f.; p. 96) referred to this passage as a parallel to the Galenic statement. The tradition which Diogenes follows is ascribed to the early Peripatos by Diels (H. Diels–W. Kranz, Die Fragmente d. Vorsokratiker, 1934⁵, 58 B 1a). For the similarity of such views with theories of Philolaus (44 A 27 [Diels-Kranz]), cf. in general M. Wellmann, Hermes, LIV, 1919, pp. 232 ff.

[40] Deichgräber, op. cit., p. 37, n. 38, has stated that opposition to abortion is in line with certain philosophical ideas, without saying, however, which ideas these are. As his only reference he quotes Phocylides, ll. 184-5. But this poem was written by a Hellenistic Jew at the beginning of the Christian era, cf. W. Christ–W. Schmid, Geschichte d. griechischen Literatur, II⁶, 1920, pp. 621 f. Concerning the general importance of the agreement between Pythagorean and Jewish-Christian theories, cf. Dölger, op. cit., p. 23, who refers to Philo and Josephus, cf. also below, pp. 63 f.

[41] Cf. in general 58 D 8, pp. 476, 7 ff.; 477, 7 ff. [Diels-Kranz] (from Aristoxenus), and Zeller, op. cit., III, 1, p. 143, n. 3; cf. ibid. I, 1⁵, p. 462, n. 2. Cf. especially p. 476, 4 [Diels-Kranz]: ὑπελάμβανον δ', ὡς ἔοικεν, ἐκεῖνοι οἱ ἄνδρες περιαιρεῖν μὲν δεῖν τάς τε παρὰ φύσιν γεννήσεις καὶ τὰς μεθ' ὕβρεως γιγνομένας, καταλιμπάνειν δὲ τῶν κατὰ φύσιν τε καὶ μετὰ σωφροσύνης γινομένων τὰς ἐπὶ τεκνοποιίᾳ σώφρονί τε καὶ νομίμῳ γινομένας. It is sometimes claimed that Aristoxenus' report is reminiscent of Platonic ethics, cf. E. Rohde, Kleine Schriften, II, 1901, p. 162. Yet in regard to

to them were more than future members of a community or citizens of a state. It was considered man's duty to beget children so as to leave behind in his own place another worshipper of the gods.[42] With such convictions how could the Pythagoreans ever allow abortive remedies to be applied? How could they fail to condemn practices of this kind, so common among their compatriots?[43]

It stands to reason, then, that the Hippocratic Oath, in its abortion-clause no less than in its prohibition of suicide, echoes Pythagorean doctrines. In no other stratum of Greek opinion were such views held or proposed in the same spirit of uncompromising austerity.[44] When the physician, after having foresworn ever to give poison or abortive remedies, adds: "In purity and holiness I will guard my life and my art," it must be the purity and holiness of the "Pythagorean way of life"[45] to which he dedicates himself.

B

The General Rules of the Ethical Code

The question now arises whether what is true of certain of the ethical clauses of the Hippocratic Oath is true of all of them, in other words, whether the whole medical code is in agreement with Pythagorean philosophy. By this latter term I mean Pythagoreanism as it was understood in the 4th century B. C. It is to this form of the dogma that the rules discussed so far were related, and it seems fair

the matter under discussion Plato's views certainly were more lax than those of the Pythagoreans, cf. *Laws*, VIII, 841 d, and above, p. 16.

[42] Cf. 58 C 4, p. 465, 5 [Diels-Kranz]: . . . ὅτι δεῖ τεκνοποιεῖσθαι ἕνεκα τοῦ καταλιπεῖν ἕτερον ἀνθ' ἑαυτοῦ θεῶν θεραπευτήν; cf. also *ibid.*, p. 464, 22. These statements are considered by Diels to be part of the old Pythagorean *Symbola*. Plato, *Laws*, VI, 773 e; 776 b, agrees with the point of view of the Pythagoreans, much as he deviates from it in other passages.

[43] Reinach, *op. cit.*, p. 321, on the evidence of a very late Orphic fragment, claims that it was the Orphics who favored rejection of abortion. But his argument is no more cogent in this respect than it is in regard to suicide, cf. above, p. 15, n. 33.

[44] It seems worth pointing out that both stipulations of the *Oath* show some affinity with ideas credited especially to Philolaus, cf. above, p. 15; p. 17, n. 39, and below, p. 57. This philosopher lived for some time in Thebes. It is therefore hardly by chance that this city alone in late sources is said to have had laws against suicide, cf. above, p. 13, n. 24. It seems probable that the well-known theory of the famous philosopher was projected into the legislation of Thebes.

[45] Cf. Plato, *Republic*, X, 600 b: . . . Πυθαγόρειον τρόπον . . . τοῦ βίου.

THE ETHICAL CODE 19

to assume that the rest of the stipulations, if at all influenced by Pythagorean thinking, correspond to the same concept of Pythagoreanism. At any rate, wherever I shall speak of Pythagorean doctrines without qualification, it is neither the teachings of the "historical" Pythagoras, nor those of the later so-called Neo-Pythagoreans which I have in mind, but rather those theories and beliefs which writers of the 4th century B. C., men like Plato, Aristotle and their pupils, attributed to Pythagoras and his followers.[46]

To start, then, with the analysis of that section of the ethical code which deals with the treatment of diseases proper:[47] here mention is made of diet, drugs and cutting. In a more technical language, medicine is viewed as comprising dietetics, pharmacology and surgery. Consequently those matters are discussed which seem most important for the attitude of the physician within these three departments of his art.[48] Now a division of medicine into these branches is not unusual and in itself is not indicative of any particular medical or philosophical school. But, according to Aristoxenus, the Pythagoreans were among those who accepted this particular classification of medicine; moreover, the sequence of the various parts of the

[46] For the very complex Pythagoras problem, cf. e. g. F. Ueberweg- K. Praechter, *Die Philosophie des Altertums*[12], 1926, pp. 61 ff. That the various forms of Pythagoreanism, especially the earliest doctrine and that of the 4th century B. C., must be sharply distinguished admits of no doubt after the studies of E. Frank, *Plato u. d. sogenannten Pythagoreer*, 1923. To him I am also indebted for his advice in many a controversial matter discussed in this paper.

[47] The ethical code can be divided into two parts of which the first (cf. above, p. 2, 12-18) outlines rules for the healing of diseases, whereas the second (cf. above, p. 2, 19-24) regulates the physician's behavior in all matters indirectly connected with the treatment, such as his relations to the patient, to the patient's family, and so forth.

[48] Cf. e. g. Münzer, *Münchener Medizinische Wochenschrift*, 1919, p. 309; Körner, *op. cit.*, p. 7. Concerning poison and abortive remedies as drugs, cf. above, p. 6. The οὐ τεμέω-clause, whatever its meaning (cf. below, pp. 24 ff.), certainly refers to surgical procedure. Deichgräber, *op. cit.*, p. 31, translates διαιτήματα with "Verordnungen" and adds, n. 24: "... eigentlich handelt es sich ... um diätetische Verordnungen." There is no reason for taking the word to mean anything but "diätetische Verordnungen"; moreover, whatever may be understood by this term, the application of drugs cannot be covered by it, cf. below, p. 23. Therefore Körner, *op. cit.*, p. 11, is not right in saying: "... Diät ... es ist also das gesamte Heilverfahren gemeint;" he himself admits that διαιτήματα does not include drugs.

healing art in the Pythagorean doctrine is the same as it is in the Hippocratic Oath, dietetics coming first, pharmacology next, surgery last.[49]

In detail, the physician is asked to use dietetic means to the advantage of his patients as his judgment and capacity permit; moreover he is enjoined to keep them from mischief and injustice.[50] That the doctor's dietetic prescriptions should be given to help the patient is an obvious truth. It is the goal of all good craftsmanship to seek the best for the object with which the craftsman is concerned. Every ancient physician would have subscribed to such a formulation.[51] It suffices to say that the Pythagorean physicians did not feel differently, for this school acknowledged the useful and the advantageous as second among the aims of human endeavor.[52]

But what exactly is meant by the promise to keep the patient from mischief and injustice? Can this really imply, as some scholars have

---

[49] Littré, op. cit., IV, p. 622, says that such a division is known only since the time of Herophilus, cf. Celsus, I, 1; cf. also below, p. 29. As a matter of fact, it is attributed to the Pythagoreans by Aristoxenus, cf. 58 D 1, p. 467, 5 ff. [Diels-Kranz]. Since this passage is fundamental for the interpretation of Pythagorean medicine, and the most extensive one preserved, I shall give it here in full: τῆς δὲ ἰατρικῆς μάλιστα μὲν ἀποδέχεσθαι τὸ διαιτητικὸν εἶδος καὶ εἶναι ἀκριβεστάτους ἐν τούτῳ· καὶ πειρᾶσθαι πρῶτον μὲν καταμανθάνειν σημεῖα συμμετρίας ποτῶν τε καὶ σίτων καὶ ἀναπαύσεως. ἔπειτα περὶ αὐτῆς τῆς κατασκευῆς τῶν προσφερομένων σχεδὸν πρώτους ἐπιχειρῆσαί τε πραγματεύεσθαι καὶ διορίζειν. ἅψασθαι δὲ [χρὴ] καὶ καταπλασμάτων ἐπὶ πλείω τοὺς Πυθαγορείους τῶν ἔμπροσθεν, τὰ δὲ περὶ τὰς φαρμακείας ἧττον δοκιμάζειν, αὐτῶν δὲ τούτων τοῖς πρὸς τὰς ἑλκώσεις μάλιστα χρῆσθαι, ⟨τὰ δὲ⟩ περὶ τὰς τομάς τε καὶ καύσεις ἥκιστα πάντων ἀποδέχεσθαι.

[50] Cf. above, p. 2, 12-13. Littré, op. cit., IV, p. 631, says: "Je m'abstiendrai de tout mal et de toute injustice;" the same meaning is given by F. Adams, The Genuine Works of Hippocrates, II, 1886, p. 279, and also by Jones, op. cit., p. 9. But εἴρξειν is transitive; it cannot possibly refer to the physician himself, cf. Daremberg, op. cit., p. 8, n. 6, with regard to Littré's translation: "Le text se refuse absolument à ce sens." With Daremberg agree Deichgräber, op. cit., p. 31, and Körner, op. cit., p. 11. The latter quite rightly points out that in Littré's interpretation the words are a mere duplication of what is said later on, cf. below, p. 32.

[51] Cf. e. g. Ps. Hippocrates, Epidemiae, I, 11, quoted above p. 11, n. 18, where the aim of medicine is defined as "to help or not to harm."

[52] For the Pythagoreans, cf. p. 474, 36 ff. [Diels-Kranz] (Aristoxenus). The συμφέρον and ὠφέλιμον were second in rank to the καλόν and εὔσχημον. It is worth noting that in later Pythagorean tradition Pythagoras himself is said to have come into this world for the benefit (εἰς ὠφέλειαν) of mankind, and to have philosophized and acted to this end (ἐπ' ὠφελείᾳ), cf. Iamblichus, De Vita Pythagorica, 30; 162; 222.

suggested, that the physician shall enforce his treatment even against the resistance or indifference of his patient's family?[53] It is true, interference of others may occur and the physician may have to contend with it, but this happens rarely, too seldom indeed to have been considered in the medical code. Moreover, while mischief may be done to the sick by his friends, why should he suffer injustice from those who wish him well?[54] And why should this danger be any greater in regard to the dietetic treatment of diseases for which case alone mention is made of it, than it would be in regard to everything else the physician may prescribe or do? No, it can scarcely be protection from the wrong done by others that the physician vows to give to his patients. But since it can neither be protection from the wrong which he himself may do,[55] one must conclude that he promises to guard his patients against the evil which they may suffer through themselves. That men by nature are liable to inflict upon themselves injustice and mischief, and that this tendency becomes apparent in all matters concerned with their regimen, this is indeed an axiom of Pythagorean dietetics.[56]

The Pythagoreans defined all bodily appetites as propensities of the soul, as a craving for the presence or absence of certain things. Most of these appetites they considered as acquired or created by

[53] Cf. Körner, op. cit., p. 11: "Der Arzt soll es (sc. the treatment) auch durchsetzen gegenüber Gleichgültigkeit oder Widerspenstigkeit der Umgebung des Kranken. Nur so kann es verstanden werden, wenn der Schwörende im Anschluss an die Anordnung des Heilverfahrens verspricht, Gefährdung und Schädigung vom Kranken abzuwehren." Daremberg, op. cit., p. 8, n. 6, compares the statement with the Hippocratic ὠφελεῖν ἢ μὴ βλάπτειν (cf. above, p. 20, n. 51), but here it is certainly the physician himself who is supposed not to do any harm, and yet, as Daremberg has shown (cf. above, p. 20, n. 51), this is not what is meant in the Oath. The other interpreters are silent about the implications of the words in question.

[54] Körner, loc. cit., very significantly translates δήλησις and ἀδικίη with "Gefährdung und Schädigung," terms which do not bring out the full impact of the Greek words.

[55] Cf. above p. 20, n. 50.

[56] In order to gain a picture of Pythagorean medicine the evidence must be put together bit by bit. Modern literature on the subject is scarce. The outline given by I. Schumacher, Antike Medizin, I, 1940, pp. 34 ff., proves unsatisfactory because here the sources are not properly evaluated. Of great importance are the study of the doctrine of κάθαρσις by E. Howald, Hermes, LIV, 1919, pp. 203 ff., and the discussion of some of the fragments by A. E. Taylor, A Commentary on Plato's Timaeus, 1928, pp. 629 ff.

men themselves, and therefore they thought human desires were to be watched closely and to be scrutinized severely. As a natural process they acknowledged only that the body should take in an appropriate amount of food and should be cleansed again appropriately after it had been filled. To overload oneself with superfluous food and drink was regarded as an acquired inclination of the soul.[57]

But unfortunately all bodily passions have the tendency to increase indefinitely. Of themselves they become "idle, irreverent, harmful and licentious,"[58] as one can readily see in those who are in the position to live according to their wishes. In order to live right from early youth on, one must learn to hold in contempt those things that are "idle and superfluous."[59] It is necessary, therefore, to select the nourishment of the body with great caution, to determine its quality and quantity most carefully, a supreme wisdom entrusted to the physicians.[60]

This is the Pythagorean doctrine concerning the regimen of the healthy. It is clear, I think, that in such a theory bodily and psychic factors are blended in a peculiar way. At the same time there is a moral element involved: unhealthy desire is uncontrolled desire; a decision is to be made between those appetites which ought to be satisfied and those which ought to be disregarded. Moreover, the Pythagorean teaching, in a strange manner, insists on negative instances. Not that alone which one does is important; that which one does not do, or is not allowed to do, carries just as much consequence. Right living is brought about not only, not even primarily, through positive actions, but rather through avoidance of those steps that are dangerous, through the repression of insatiable desires which if left to themselves would cause damage.[61]

The same consideration for body and soul, the same combination

---

[57] Cf. 58 D 8, p. 474, 40-p. 475, 8 [Diels-Kranz] (from Aristoxenus).

[58] Ibid., p. 475, 14-17: μάλιστα δ' εἶναι κατανοῆσαι τάς τε ματαίους καὶ τὰς βλαβερὰς καὶ τὰς περιέργους καὶ τὰς ὑβριστικὰς τῶν ἐπιθυμιῶν παρὰ τῶν ἐν ἐξουσίαις ἀναστρεφομένων γινομένας.

[59] Ibid., p. 475, 11: . . . ἀφέξονται δὲ τῶν ματαίων τε καὶ περιέργων ἐπιθυμιῶν . . . .

[60] Cf. ibid., p. 475, 29-33; for ancient theories concerning the dietetics of the healthy in general, cf. L. Edelstein, Die Antike, VII, 1931, pp. 255 ff.

[61] A late Pythagorean poem still defines the right measure to be applied in matters concerning health, the μέτρον, as ὃ μή σ' ἀνιήσει, that which will not harm you (Carmen Aureum, l. 34); for the date of this poem, cf. below p. 33, n. 105.

of precepts and prohibitions seems to be characteristic of the Pythagorean treatment of diseases. Most illnesses, in the opinion of these philosophers, are due to opulent living; too much food is consumed which cannot be digested properly, and thus extravagance destroys the body, just as it destroys wealth.[62] If health, the retention of the form, changes into disease, the destruction of the form, the body needs purification through medicine, just as the sick soul needs purification through music.[63] The physician in such a case must give assistance by changing the patient's regimen. He must use dietetical means, as the Hippocratic Oath says.[64] In choosing them he will be intent on his patient's benefit according to the best of his judgment and ability. Whatever he prescribes, as a true follower of Pythagoras he will remember one fundamental truth: everything that is given to the body creates a certain disposition of the soul. Men in general, though they are aware of the fact that some things, such as wine, may suddenly bring about a striking change in a person's behavior, do not apprehend that every kind of food or drink causes a certain mental habit, slight as the variations may be. But the physician

[62] Cf. Diodorus, X, 7, 1: ὅτι παρεκάλει τὴν λιτότητα ζηλοῦν· τὴν γὰρ πολυτέλειαν ἅμα τάς τε οὐσίας τῶν ἀνθρώπων διαφθείρειν καὶ τὰ σώματα. Aristoxenus expresses the same idea by speaking of human beings as a ποικιλώτατον . . . γένος κατὰ τὸ τῶν ἐπυθυμιῶν πλῆθος (p. 475, 18-19 [Diels-Kranz]). A similar view is ascribed to Pythagoras himself by Apollonius, cf. Iamblichus, De Vita Pythagorica, 218; cf. also Rohde, op. cit., p. 164. I owe this reference to Schumacher, op. cit., p. 56.

[63] Cf. 58 C 3, p. 463, 26 [Diels-Kranz]: ὑγίειαν τὴν τοῦ εἴδους διαμονήν, νόσον τὴν τούτου φθοράν (from Aristotle). This concept can be elaborated by comparing the definition of health as harmony, the proper attunement of the body, ibid., p. 451, 11 (early Peripatetic tradition), and by referring to Alcmaeon's definition of health as ἰσονομία of the qualities, and of disease as μοναρχία of one quality (24 B4 [Diels-Kranz]; note also the expression φθοροποιόν). For medicine as κάθαρσις cf. ibid., 58 D 1, p. 468, 19 ff.: ὅτι οἱ Πυθαγορικοί, ὡς ἔφη Ἀριστόξενος, καθάρσει ἐχρῶντο τοῦ μὲν σώματος διὰ τῆς ἰατρικῆς, τῆς δὲ ψυχῆς διὰ τῆς μουσικῆς; cf. Howald, op. cit., p. 203.

[64] That in these instances the prescription of diet is the correct way of treatment follows from the alleged cause of the diseases, cf. above, pp. 21 f. This is also confirmed by the fact that dietetics was the principal treatment given by the Pythagoreans, as Aristoxenus says, cf. below, p. 29. The methods outlined in the Platonic Timaeus, a Pythagorean dialogue if there is any, are identical. Plato uses almost the same words: διὸ παιδαγωγεῖν δεῖ διαίταις . . . (89 c); Littré, op. cit., IV, p. 622, also referred to this passage in explanation of the Hippocratic δίαιται; cf. Körner, op. cit., p. 11.

knows that—his art primarily consists in this knowledge.[65] Consequently, he must see to it that the soul of the sick, through a wrong
diet, does not fall into "idle, irreverent, harmful and licentious passions." Since he acts according to this principle when assisting the
healthy,[66] he must certainly do likewise when treating the sick. Or
in the words of the Hippocratic Oath: the physician must protect
his patient from the mischief and injustice which he may inflict
upon himself if his diet is not properly chosen.[67] He must be a
physician of the soul no less than of the body; he must not overlook
the moral implications of his actions, nor even the negative indices
to be watched; for the regimen followed by a person concerns both
his bodily and his psychic constitution.[68]

The rules concerning dietetics, then, agree with Pythagoreanism,
in fact they acquire meaning only if seen in the light of Pythagorean
teaching. That the pharmacological precepts, the stipulations concerning poison and abortion, are Pythagorean in origin has already
been demonstrated.[69] It remains to be shown that the laws laid down
for surgery, too, are most easily understandable on the theory that
they are founded on Pythagorean doctrine.

The physician vows: "I will not use the knife either on sufferers
from stone, but I will give place to such as are craftsmen therein";
this at least is the most common rendering of the words in question.[70] Supposing that it be correct, what should be the reason for

[65] Cf. p. 475, 25-33 [Diels-Kranz]: διὸ δὴ καὶ μεγάλης σοφίας ⟨δεῖσθαι⟩ τὸ κατανοῆ-
σαί τε καὶ συνιδεῖν, ποίοις τε καὶ πόσοις δεῖ χρῆσθαι πρὸς τὴν τροφήν. εἶναι δὲ ταύτην
τὴν ἐπιστήμην τὸ μὲν ἐξ ἀρχῆς Ἀπόλλωνός τε καὶ Παιῶνος, ὕστερον δὲ τῶν περὶ τὸν
Ἀσκληπιόν (from Aristoxenus).

[66] Cf. above, pp. 21 f.

[67] Mischief (δήλησις) obviously is identical with what Aristoxenus calls βλαβεραὶ
ἐπιθυμίαι; injustice (ἀδικία) is a concept that is implied by ὑβριστικαὶ ἐπιθυμίαι;
cf. above, p. 22.

[68] Note that Plato in the Timaeus, 87 d, says that nothing is more dangerous
than the ἀμετρία . . . ψυχῆς . . . πρὸς σῶμα; later on he states that most of the
so-called physicians are deceived in their treatment because they seek the cause of
the disease in the body, whereas in reality it is to be found in the soul (88 a).

[69] Cf. above p. 18. What the Pythagoreans understood by pharmacology and
how they made use of it can be concluded from Aristoxenus' statement, quoted
above, p. 20, n. 49. For more details cf. below, pp. 29 f.

[70] For the text, cf. above, p. 2, 17-18; for the translation, cf. Jones, op. cit., p. 11
(but cf. below, p. 28, n. 84); Littré, op. cit., IV, p. 631; Daremberg, op. cit., p. 5;

the prohibition here pronounced? The treatment of stone-diseases by operation, in Greek medicine, seems to have been an old-established procedure; at any rate, since the rise of Alexandrian medicine, such an operation was performed throughout the centuries.[71] Why then is it forbidden in the Oath?

From the Renaissance down to the 19th century there was only one answer to this question: 'the Oath in the clause concerning lithotomy intends to draw a line between the practice of internal medicine and that of surgery. This separation, it was added, is introduced because surgery was held to be beneath the dignity of the physician.[72] With finer historical judgment, Littré rejected this generally accepted view. He pointed out that the ancient practitioner was a surgeon as well as a physician and considered the interpretation current before his time to be influenced by modern prejudices; but he had to admit that if this were so the statement seemed to defy explanation.[73] Indeed if the words in question do not have the meaning usually presumed, what else could they signify?

Littré with great hesitation and caution intimated that the stumbling block could perhaps be removed by the assumption that the Oath does not refer to lithotomy at all, but to castration. Some modern scholars have accepted this suggestion. For moral reasons

Pétrequin, op. cit., I, p. 187; J. Hirschberg, Vorlesungen über hippokratische Heilkunde, 1922, p. 27; Körner, op. cit., p. 12.

[71] Littré, op. cit., IV, pp. 615 ff., has argued very convincingly that the operation must have been known since an early period because in Ps. Hippocrates, De Morbis, I, 6, diagnosis of the disease by means of a catheter is referred to as part of good craftsmanship. From Celsus, VII, 26, it follows that in his time great improvements in technique were made. Meges and Ammonius whom he mentions probably lived in the 1st century A.D.; cf. Hirschberg, op. cit., p. 31; but the operation was certainly performed before; cf. Littré's interpretation of the passage, op. cit., I, p. 342. For lithotomy in late centuries, cf. Ps. Galen, Introductio (Galen, XIV, p. 787 K.). Hirschberg, op. cit., p. 32, believes that the Alexandrian physicians were the first to practice lithotomy, but this assumption he derives from the interdiction of this operation in the Hippocratic Oath which he considers a very old document (cf. ibid., p. 27). Such an argumentation, of course, is not cogent, since it is precisely the date of the Oath which has not been established so far.

[72] Cf. e. g. Th. Zwinger, Hippocratis Opera, 1579, p. 59. Cf. also I. Cornarius, Hippocratis Opera, 1558, p. 8; P. Memmius and J. Fabricius in their commentaries on the Oath, published in 1577 and 1614 respectively. Cf. in general Körner, op. cit., pp. 14 ff.; but cf. also below, p. 27, n. 80.

[73] Cf. Littré, op. cit., IV, pp. 616-17.

they have said the physician abhorred such a treatment.[74] I shall not repeat the argument that has been brought forward before: to reject castration on moral grounds and yet to leave it to others would be "like compounding a felony, if not something worse."[75] Although from a linguistic point of view it is not impossible to understand the text as referring to castration, such a rendering is not consistent with the subject matter. For it is not attested that the ancients ever thought of applying castration as treatment of stone-diseases.[76] The sentence under discussion, therefore, must concern lithotomy, not castration.

Now some scholars, recognizing the fact that the Oath refers to lithotomy, contend that impotence was likely to result from the operation and that the physician recoiled from this risk — "it was against his liking"; "a higher concept of his profession" is supposed to have determined his renunciation of operative treatment by which he lost a good source of making money.[77] But such an inter-

[74] Cf. Littré, op. cit., IV, p. 620 (with reference to R. Moreau, a physician of the 17th century; cf. ibid., p. 618); Th. Gomperz, Griechische Denker, I⁴, 1922, p. 231; in general S. Nittis, The Hippocratic Oath in reference to lithotomy, A new interpretation with historical notes on castration, Bulletin of the History of Medicine, VII, 1939, pp. 719 ff.

[75] Cf. Jones, op. cit., p. 48; cf. also Körner, op. cit., pp. 12 ff. Nittis being aware of the difficulties pointed out by Jones and Körner tries to evade them by translating ἐκχωρήσω etc. by "I will keep apart from men engaging in this deed" (op. cit., p. 721). He thinks that this might be the meaning of the verb ἐκχωρήσω, but he is unable to adduce any evidence for such a usage: the meaning of χωρέω of course does not prove anything in regard to that of ἐκχωρέω, and ἀποστήσομαι to which Nittis refers as a parallel has exactly the sense of ἐκχωρέω as it is usually taken. How inappropriate Nittis' rendering is, one can easily conclude from an old variant of the Oath: οὔτ' ἐμοῖσι δὲ οὔτ' ἄλλοισι ἐκχωρήσω . . . (Jones, op. cit., p. 19).

[76] Nittis who has carefully investigated the history of castration comes to the following conclusion (op. cit., p. 728): "Castration . . . was . . . probably practiced for the cure and prevention of diseases. Lithiasis is not mentioned directly by any writer as one of the diseases preventable by castration . . . ." In view of the fact that castration cannot be meant here, it is unnecessary to discuss the many emendations proposed to facilitate this interpretation, cf. Hirschberg, op. cit., p. 29. To rectify an assertion which has frequently been made, I wish to mention at least that ancient physicians are known to have practiced castration for purposes other than medical, cf. Littré, op. cit., IV, pp. 618 ff.

[77] Cf. Hirschberg, op. cit., p. 30: "Eine solche Operation ging der Gilde gegen den Strich." As he says, Wilamowitz and Diels accepted his view. So does Deichgräber, op. cit., p. 37, who writes: "Auch hier erhebt sich der Eid über die Sphäre der gewöhnlichen Handelsweise zu einer höheren Auffassung und wieder wird dem praktischen Arzte eine Erwerbsquelle verschlossen."

pretation can hardly be correct. To emphasize it once more: if the physician for moral reasons refuses to undertake the operation, he cannot possibly say in the same breath that he " will give place to such as are craftsmen therein." [78] The author of the Oath in other instances does not shrink from forbidding unconditionally what is held immoral or objectionable: when prohibiting the use of poison and of abortive remedies he does not say that the application of these drugs should be left to somebody else. The concession made in regard to lithotomy proves beyond doubt that the operation as such is not condemned: the performance of lithotomy, though not considered the business of the physician, is left to others for whom apparently it is judged legitimate.[79]

If this is true it seems to follow that lithotomy was to be given into the hands of specialists who were better able to do the job, that the Oath requires the physician to keep strictly within the limits of his own knowledge and recognize the superior skill of others who in some instances could be of greater help to his patients.[80] Such an explanation again leads into great difficulties. To be sure, specialization in certain operations or diseases of certain organs was known in antiquity. The stone-disease may have been one of these illnesses; lithotomy may have been practiced by craftsmen who were experts in this specific operation.[81] But lithotomy as performed in antiquity was not a more daring operation than many another which the general practitioner undertook without hesitation. Why then should the physician acknowledge his own limitations in this par-

[78] Cf. above, p. 24.

[79] Incidentally, it is not attested that in the opinion of the ancients lithotomy could injure the procreative faculty, cf. Hirschberg's discussion of the medical aspect of the problem, *op. cit.*, pp. 30 ff., especially the passages from Celsus and Paulus of Aegina, *ibid.*, p. 32.

[80] Cf. Körner, *op. cit.*, pp. 15 ff. A very similar interpretation has been proposed by J. H. Meibom, *Hippocratis Jus Jurandum*, 1643, p. 163.

[81] The question of specialists in antiquity has been widely discussed. That from Alexandrian times on medicine became specialized can hardly be doubted. In Rome specialization in certain diseases reached a climax. Nothing definite is known about the classical period. In spite of Cicero's emphatic statement that Hippocrates still mastered the whole range of medical knowledge (*De Oratore*, III, 33) it is hard to believe that in the Hippocratic period specialization was unknown (contrary to Littré, *op. cit.*, IV, p. 615, n. 1, who follows A. Andreae, *Zur ältesten Geschichte der Augenheilkunde*, 1841); the material is too scanty to admit a decision of the issue.

ticular case?[82] If moderation on his part is the general issue, why is he not asked to forego the treatment of all diseases for which the ancients had specialists? It is true, a distinction is made in the Oath between that which the physician should do and that which he should leave to others. But this division is recommended only in regard to lithotomy, and it has to be understood with reference to this particular instance.

There is no way out of the dilemma! The words must mean what in the opinion of all early interpreters they seemed to mean: lithotomy is here excluded because the performance of operations is held to be incompatible with the physician's craft, and by the one example given the Oath intends to exclude surgery in general from the field of the physician. It is possible that originally more operations were named as forbidden, that these references are missing only in the preserved text. But such a hypothesis cannot be verified.[83] It is more probable, however, that the statement as it stands is intact but in itself carries broader implications. For instead of translating "I will not use the knife either on sufferers from stone," it is equally well possible to translate "I will not use the knife, not even on sufferers from stone."[84] This would signify that the physician

---

[82] For operations performed by general practitioners, cf. Littré, *op. cit.*, IV, p. 617. That other operations made were more dangerous than lithotomy (contrary to Körner, *op. cit.*, p. 15) has been emphasized by Hirschberg, *op. cit.*, p. 30, who also stresses the fact that the ancient writers do not speak of an especially high mortality rate in this instance.

[83] Körner, *op. cit.*, n. 16, mentions the possibility of a lacuna after οὐ τεμέω δέ; cf. also *C. M. G.*, I, 1, p. 4, 19: post δέ lacunam statuit Diels (though for other reasons; cf. Hirschberg, *op. cit.*, p. 30). Deichgräber, *op. cit.*, n. 11, considers such an assumption unnecessary.

[84] Jones is the only one who has strongly emphasized the possibility of such a rendering. Moreover he has stressed the great difference in meaning that the two translations involve (*op. cit.*, pp. 46-47; cf. also *ibid.*, p. 11, n. 1, and Hippocrates, I, pp. 293 ff. [Loeb]); cf. also Nittis, *op. cit.*, p. 720, who goes so far as to say that the usual translation of the words is grammatically incorrect. I am not sure that in this respect he is right, but I do prefer the other rendering. Deichgräber, *op. cit.*, n. 11, says of the crucial words: "οὐδέ verstärkt die Negation wie Z. 15 (*sc.* after οὐ δώσω δέ); μήν beteuert, wie oft gerade in Eidschwüren und Versprechen." But in the passage quoted by Deichgräber, οὐδέ is used, not οὐδέ μήν; this fact is indicative of a difference in meaning. For οὐδέ μήν in the sense of intensification (not even), cf. Kühner-Gerth, *Griechische Grammatik*, II, 2, § 502, 4 b, p. 137. Cf. also the old Latin translation (Jones, *op. cit.*, p. 37): non incidam autem neque lapiditatem patientes; another translation (*op. cit.*, p. 35) corresponds to the rendering of most modern interpreters.

directly renounces operative surgery altogether. He will not resort to it even in the case of that disease which more than any other, according to the testimony of the ancients, drove men to suicide.[85] The prohibition could not be formulated in more emphatic and solemn words.

Whatever rendering is chosen, the statement under discussion enjoins a separation of medicine and surgery. Driven back to this interpretation which no doubt is drastically at variance with reality, one feels almost inclined to say with Littré that such an explanation must be rejected, and that consequently the motive for the interdiction of lithotomy in the Oath remains obscure.[86] Yet this seems to be too rash a conclusion. It is true that the depreciation of surgery was foreign to ancient physicians in general.[87] It is likewise true, however, that one medical sect valued surgery less highly than dietetics and pharmacology, I mean the Pythagorean physicians. As Aristoxenus says, they believed "most of all" in dietetics; they applied poultices more liberally than did their predecessors, but "thought less" of the efficacy of drugs; "they believed least of all in using the knife and in cauterizing." [88] In other words, according to Aristoxenus, the Pythagoreans attributed different values to the various branches of medicine, and in their classification operative surgery together with cauterization was ranked lowest. If one remembers that in Aristoxenus' opinion the Pythagoreans explained most diseases as the result of unreasonable living,[89] one is at first inclined to conclude that they were mainly interested in dietetics

[85] Cf. above, p. 8, n. 9, finis.

[86] Cf. Littré, op. cit., p. 617. It is of course impossible to say with Jones, op. cit., p. 48, or K. Sprengel, Apologie des Hippokrates, I, p. 77 (cf. Littré, op. cit., I, p. 342), that the words in question are a later addition. If this statement were missing, surgery would not be referred to at all in the Oath.

[87] Cf. e. g. Littré, op. cit., IV, p. 617. A separation of surgery from internal medicine can be traced at best to Galen's time (cf. Galen, X, pp. 454-55 K.; Jones, op. cit., p. 48), that is, in the sense that physicians refused to practice surgery because they held it beneath their dignity. The study and teaching of the various branches of medicine had become specialized long before, cf. Celsus, Introductio, 9; cf. also above, p. 27, n. 81.

[88] Cf. 58 D 1 [Diels-Kranz] (quoted above, p. 20, n. 49); cf. Porphyry, Vita Pythagorae, 22: φυγαδευτέον πάσῃ μηχανῇ καὶ περικοπτέον πυρὶ καὶ σιδήρῳ καὶ μηχαναῖς παντοίαις ἀπὸ μὲν σώματος νόσον . . . (Aristoxenus = Fr. 8 [Müller]).

[89] Cf. above, pp. 20 ff.

and pharmacology, because these were the more appropriate means of treatment. Still this can hardly be the whole truth. For Plato in the *Timaeus*, when outlining the Pythagorean treatment of diseases, does not mention cutting or cauterizing at all, though he agrees with Aristoxenus in placing the importance of pharmacology after that of dietetics.[90] Evidently, then, there must have been Pythagoreans who refused to apply any surgical means of treatment which were otherwise so universally used in Greek medicine. This inference from the Platonic *Timaeus* seems quite certain though no express statement to this effect is preserved.[91]

It is most likely that Aristoxenus' report is one of his typical attempts to reconcile the rigorous Pythagorean attitude with the demands of common sense and the exigencies of daily life: such compromises he introduces in many instances where other sources attest the uncompromising attitude of the Pythagoreans.[92] Seen

[90] Cf. *Timaeus*, 87 c ff.; esp. 89 d.

[91] Note how in contrast to the passage in the *Timaeus*, Plato in the *Republic*, III, 405 c ff., defines medicine as the art which should deal with drugs or cauterization and cutting, whereas the pedagogics of dietetic medicine is rejected (406 d). It can hardly be by chance that Plato omits a reference to cutting and cauterization in the *Timaeus*. In K. Sprengel– I. Rosenbaum, *Versuch einer pragmatischen Geschichte der Arzneikunde*, I, 1846, p. 251, it is said: " Der schneidenden und brennenden Werkzeuge enthielt er (*sc.* Pythagoras) sich gänzlich," but the only testimony adduced is the fragment of Aristoxenus (cf. above, p. 20, n. 49). J. F. K. Hecker, *Geschichte der Heilkunde*, I, 1822, p. 77, claims that: " . . . die Pythagorische Arzneikunst sich viel mit äusseren Mitteln beschäftigte, von der kühnern Chirurgie aber ganz entfernt blieb." He does not give any proof for this assertion. The more recent books on Pythagorean medicine do not discuss the problem at all. For the modern it may be difficult to imagine a medical art without surgery in the strict sense of the word (the treatment of fractures and so forth is of course not curtailed by the prohibition of operative surgery). Yet in antiquity popular opposition to " cutting and cauterization" was strong indeed. Cf. *e. g.* Plato, *Gorgias*, 456 b, and the parallels collected in Stallbaum's commentary *ad locum*. The attitude of the ancients never changed in this respect; cf. the most impressive statement of Scribonius Largus, *Compositiones*, p. 2, ll. 3 ff. [Helmreich]: " . . . siquidem verum est antiquos herbis ac radicibus earum corporis vitia curasse, quia timidum genus mortalium inter initia non facile se ferro ignique comittebat. quod etiam nunc plerique faciunt, ne dicam omnes, et nisi magna conpulsi necessitate speque ipsius salutis non patiuntur sibi fieri, quae sane vix sunt toleranda."

[92] Note *e. g.* Aristoxenus' denial of the contention that Pythagoras refrained from all bloody sacrifices, p. 101, 13 ff. [Diels-Kranz], or his claim that he did not reject beans as nourishment, *ibid.*, p. 101, 19 ff., whereas others see in this prohibition a means of purification, *ibid.*, p. 463, 10 (Aristotle), p. 451, 15 ff. (early

from this angle, the stipulation of the Oath appears as another compromise, more lenient and at the same time more rigid than that reported by Aristoxenus: the use of cauterization obviously is allowed, operative surgery is completely eliminated. On the other hand, the Pythagorean physician will allow others to help his patient in his extremity. The stipulation against operating is valid only for him who has dedicated himself to a holy life. The Pythagoreans recognized that men in general could not observe any elaborate rules of purity; in this fact they saw no argument against that which they considered right for themselves. To give place to another craftsman, especially in such instances where the patient might fall prey to a sinful temptation,[93] certainly was a duty demanded by philanthropy, by commiseration with those who suffered.[94]

But why should the Pythagorean have avoided the use of the knife? The answer can only be a conjecture: he who believed that bloody sacrifices should not be offered to the gods and saw in them a defilement of divine purity could well believe that he himself would be defiled in his purity and holiness by using the knife in bloody operations.[95] However that may be, it is only in connection with

Peripatos). P. Corssen, *Rheinisches Museum*, LXVII, 1912, p. 258, intimated that Aristoxenus in his interpretation of Pythagorean philosophy is inclined to make the doctrine appear less rigid than it is portrayed by others. Cf. moreover Ueberweg-Praechter, *op. cit.*, p. 64.

[93] Cf. above, p. 8, n. 9; p. 15.

[94] Already in Peripatetic attacks on the Pythagorean way of life the question was raised how a state could be governed in which everybody followed the Pythagorean taboos. The answer was that these purity-observances were not meant to be valid for everybody; cf. Porphyry, *De Abstinentia*, I, and J. Bernays, *Theophrastos' Schrift über Frömmigkeit*, 1866, p. 13. Moreover, the Pythagorean ideal of government is that of an aristocracy with proportionally divided rights and duties, cf. M. Pohlenz, *Aus Platos Werdezeit*, 1913, p. 154, n. 1 (Dicaearchus).

[95] There is no need for an elaborate discussion of the Pythagorean rejection of bloody sacrifices in which their insistence on purity manifested itself most clearly, cf. *e. g.* Diogenes Laertius, VIII, 13, and in general Bernays, who quite rightly speaks of the "Pythagoreische Blutscheu" (*op. cit.*, p. 33); cf. also the Pythagorean objections to the drinking of wine "the blood of the earth," Corssen, *op. cit.*, pp. 246 ff. (Androcydes). For the concept of defilement, cf. such expressions as Plato, *Laws*, VI, 782 c: τοὺς τῶν θεῶν βωμοὺς αἵματι μιαίνειν; cf. also Bernays, *op. cit.*, p. 130. For purification rites in regard to the knife that is used in bloody sacrifices, cf. Bernays, *op. cit.*, p. 91. Note that Aristoxenus, according to whom surgery, though valued least, was nevertheless practiced by the Pythagoreans, denies that they offered only bloodless gifts to the gods; cf. above, p. 30, n. 92.

Pythagorean medicine that the injunction of the Hippocratic Oath, according to which operative surgery was forbidden to the physician, acquires any meaning and plausibility at all. The rules given in regard to surgery no less than those concerning dietetics and pharmacology are Pythagorean in character.[96]

Those stipulations of the Oath which deal with the medical treatment proper are finally followed by two more general provisions bearing on medical ethics in the strict sense of the word. The behavior of the physician towards his patient and the patient's family is regulated; reticence is imposed upon him in regard to whatever he may see or hear. Is it really true that in non-medical literature no parallels can be found to these postulates?[97] In my opinion these ethical rules, too, in their specific wording are understandable only in connection with Pythagorean doctrine.

As for the first vow, he who swears the Oath promises to come, into whatever house he enters, to help the sick, refraining from injustice and mischief, especially from all sexual incontinence.[98] That the physician should act for the sole purpose of assisting his patient, is a demand that seems self-evident. It certainly is as compatible with any ethical standard to which a doctor may subscribe, as it is with Pythagorean ethics.[99] It may seem equally natural that the physician is bidden to refrain from all injustice and mischief. Yet, the appropriateness of the statement does not imply that it is not in need of further explanation, be it in regard to its meaning or its motivation.[100]

Those who believe that only medical parallels can be adduced for

[96] Cf. above, pp. 19 f., where it is shown that even the sequence of dietetics, pharmacology and surgery, as given in the Oath, corresponds to the sequence of these branches of medicine in the report of Aristoxenus.

[97] Cf. Deichgräber, op. cit., p. 37: " Während sich die drei ersten Bestimmungen (sc. concerning dietetics, pharmacology, and surgery) mit ausserhalb der medizinischen Kreise und des medizinischen Bereiches geltenden Maximen vergleichen lassen, ist für diese Beschränkungen eine derartige Gegenüberstellung nicht möglich. Nur ein Vergleich mit den sonst in der hippokratischen Pflichtenlehre geltenden Anschauungen lässt sich durchführen . . ." (cf. however below, p. 33, n. 104). The other interpreters do not attempt at all to give an explanation of these rules.

[98] Cf. above, p. 2, 19-21.

[99] For the ὠφέλιμον and its rôle in Pythagoreanism, cf. above, p. 20, n. 52.

[100] Cf. Körner, op. cit., p. 16, who in his interpretation of the Oath simply says: " Das nun folgende Gelöbnis bedarf keiner Erklärung."

the stipulations of the Oath point to seemingly similar utterances in one of the so-called Hippocratic writings, the book " On the Physician."[101] Here it is stated that in his relations with the sick the doctor ought to be just, for the patients have no small dealings with their physician. They put themselves into his hands, and the physician comes in contact with women and maidens and with very precious possessions indeed; so toward all these self-control should be used.[102] I do not wish to raise the issue, whether justice is here commended for utilitarian rather than moral reasons. Nor do I emphasize the fact that only if it had a moral bent could this assertion be likened to the Oath.[103] In refutation of the argument of modern interpreters it is enough to say that the parallel referred to is by far less comprehensive and less rigorous than the statement which it is supposed to explain. The Oath, unlike the Hippocratic treatise " On the Physician," does not speak only of the avoidance of injustice, it also excludes mischief. Moreover, the Oath enjoins continence in regard to women and men alike; it stresses that the same continence must be observed towards free-born people and slaves, features that are entirely missing in the other passage.[104] A more satisfactory interpretation of the words in question, therefore, must be sought.

Now a plea for justice and continence may of course be derived from many ancient philosophical systems. As for justice, the Platonists and the Aristotelians praised its dignity no less than did the Pythagoreans.[105] But so much it is safe to claim: that the physician

[101] Cf. Deichgräber, op. cit., p. 38; but cf. also Daremberg, op. cit., p. 57.

[102] Cf. C. M. G., I, 1, p. 20, 18 ff. In my paraphrase of the very difficult passage I have partly followed Jones' translation, Hippocrates, II, p. 313 [Loeb].

[103] For the idealistic point of view consistently observed in the Oath, cf. above, p. 27, and below, p. 50. As a matter of fact the author of Περὶ ἰητροῦ is an utilitarian, cf. below, p. 37, n. 119.

[104] That this is so, is also admitted by Deichgräber, op. cit., p. 38, who adds that the attitude taken in the Oath is in agreement with that taken by certain philosophers, but he does not say who they are.

[105] For Plato and Aristotle, cf. below, p. 35, n. 112, for the Pythagoreans in general, cf. Zeller, op. cit., I, 1, p. 390. I admit that the ultimate principles of Pythagorean ethics are not well known, but this much one may venture to say: justice played an important rôle in their system. Otherwise, why should justice determine men's relation to the gods and to all other creatures in the world (cf. 58 C 4, p. 464, 8 [Diels-Kranz]; Diogenes Laertius, VIII, 23; Iamblichus, De Vita Pythagorica, 168)? Why should Pythagoras have said of salt that it should be brought to table to remind us of what is just—for salt preserves whatever it

is required to abstain from all intentional injustice and mischief—
such a formulation savors of the famous Pythagorean sayings by
which injustice and mischief are proscribed, even if committed
against animals and plants.[106] And indeed, to blend the concept of
justice with that of forbearance is characteristic of the Pythagoreans.
They abhorred violence; only if provoked by injustice would they
resort to force. In this recoiling from aggression the asceticism of
Pythagorean ethics culminated.[107] Moreover, the consequences drawn
in the Oath from the ethical standards there imposed are in strict
keeping with those principles which the Pythagoreans enforced upon
their followers. Their views on sexual matters were severer than
those of all other ancient philosophers. They alone judged sexual
relations in terms of justice, meaning thereby not that which is
forbidden or allowed by law: for the husband to be unfaithful to his
wife was considered to be unjust toward her.[108] The Pythagoreans
upheld the equality of men and women. They alone condemned
sodomy.[109] Besides, in the performance of moral duties, they did not

seasons, and it arises from the purest sources, sun and sea (cf. 58 C 3, p. 463, 27
[Diels-Kranz])? Cf. also *Carmen Aureum*, ll. 13-16. But I do not wish to lay too
much emphasis on this source, since it is of relatively late date (usually ascribed
to the first century B. C. or A. D., cf. Ueberweg-Prächter, *op. cit.*, p. 518).
Hierocles in his commentary on the *Carmen Aureum*, *Fragmenta Philosophorum
Graecorum*, ed. F. G. A. Mullach, I, 1883, p. 433, goes so far as to claim that
justice was the principal virtue of the Pythagoreans. But this is a late Neo-Platonic
re-interpretation.

[106] Cf. Diogenes Laertius, VIII, 23 (from Androcydes, cf. Corssen, *op. cit.*,
p. 258): φυτὸν ἥμερον μήτε φθίνειν μήτε σίνεσθαι, αλλὰ μηδὲ ζῷον ὃ μὴ βλάπτει
ἀνθρώπους. In other passages the words used are even more reminiscent of the
phraseology of the *Oath*, cf. Iamblichus, *De Vita Pythagorica*, 168: μήτε ἀδικεῖν
. . . μήτε φονεύειν; *ibid.*, 99: μήτε βλάπτειν μήτε φθείρειν.

[107] The renunciation of violence is a natural consequence of the Pythagorean
concept of purity and holiness. I do not think that such an ideal is to be found in
any other ethical system of the ancients. Zeller rightly ascribes to the Pythagoreans
"Gerechtigkeit und Sanftmut gegen alle Menschen," *op. cit.*, I, 1, p. 462.

[108] Cf. Ps. Aristotle, *Oeconomica*, I, 4: . . . ὑφηγεῖται δὲ [ὃ] καὶ ὁ κοινὸς νόμος,
καθάπερ οἱ Πυθαγόρειοι λέγουσιν, ὥσπερ ἱκέτιν καὶ ἀφ' ἑστίας ἠγμένην ὡς ἥκιστα δεῖν
[δοκεῖν] ἀδικεῖν· ἀδικία δὲ ἀνδρὸς αἱ θύραζε συνουσίαι γιγνόμεναι. Cf. also Diodorus,
X, 9, 3; 4; Iamblichus, *De Vita Pythagorica*, 132, and in general, above, pp. 17 f.;
cf. also Zeller, *op. cit.*, I, 1, p. 462, n. 2. How foreign such reflections are to common
Greek thought becomes apparent from Aristotle who considers adultery unjust, if
committed for gain's sake; otherwise he calls it self-indulgence, *N. E.*, 1130 a 24 ff.

[109] Concerning women in the Pythagorean school, cf. Iamblichus, *De Vita
Pythagorica*, 267; cf. Zeller, *op. cit.*, I, 1, p. 314, n. 4. As for the γεννήσεις παρὰ

discriminate between social ranks. In that respect free-born people and slaves, for the Pythagoreans, were on equal footing.[110] Everything, then, that the Oath stipulates in regard to sexual continence agrees with the tenets of Pythagorean ethics, in fact with the ideals of these philosophers alone.

Finally, as a Pythagorean postulate, the clause takes on a peculiar significance for the physician. It is justice first of all that is required from him. This virtue, to the average people, meant to live in accordance with the laws of the state.[111] To Plato, wherever he does not speak of justice in his own peculiar usage as the perfect working of the human soul in all its functions, justice was mainly a civic virtue. Aristotle tried to establish justice as a political virtue, and as one that applies to contracts and dealings in the law-courts.[112] All these aspects are also inherent in the Pythagorean concept of justice, and they certainly are of some concern for the physician. While in his direct dealings with men, in his personal contact with them and their households, it may be of less importance whether generally speaking he is a law-abiding citizen, it makes a great difference indeed, whether he is an honest man or not. It is in this sense, that even the author of the Hippocratic book " On the Phy-

φύσιν, rejected by the Pythagoreans, cf. p. 476, 4-5 [Diels-Kranz], quoted above, p. 17, n. 41. Even Plato, *Laws*, VII, 841 d, does not go as far as the Pythagoreans. For the usual Greek point of view, cf. Aristotle, *N. E.*, 1148 b 29 ff.

[110] For the Pythagorean attitude towards slaves, cf. E. Zeller–W. Nestle, *Grundriss d. Geschichte d. griech. Philosophie*[13], 1928, p. 40; but they speak only of " humane Behandlung." It would be more adequate, however, to speak of equality, though there is no express statement to this effect among the Pythagorean testimonies, cf. J. Burckhardt, *Vorträge*, 1919, p. 193. As Aristoxenus says, p. 471, 8 f. [Diels-Kranz], the true Pythagorean will not punish anybody in anger, be he slave or free. Moreover, according to Aristotle, *N. E.*, 1132 b 22, the Pythagoreans define justice as reciprocity without qualification; cf. Zeller, *op. cit.*, I, 1, p. 390, n. 1. Aristotle adds that reciprocity fits neither distributive nor rectificatory justice, meaning thereby that punishment must differ in regard to the official status of the offender. In the *Magna Moralia*, 1194 a 28, the Pythagorean definition of justice is rejected because it cannot hold good in relation to all persons, " for the same thing is not just for a domestic as for a freeman." Obviously, then, the Pythagoreans did not believe that justice should be administered differently in the case of slaves. They believed in the equality of all human beings.

[111] Cf. Aristotle, *N. E.*, V, ch. 1, where also the proverbial saying is quoted: " In justice is every virtue comprehended," 1129 b 29-30.

[112] For Plato, cf. especially *Republic*, IV, 441 c ff., and *Laws*, VI, 757 a ff.; in general cf. Zeller, *op. cit.*, II, 1[4], pp. 884-86. For Aristotle, cf. *N. E.*, V, chs. 2 ff.

sician " counsels the doctor not to infringe upon the possessions of others with whom he is doing business.[113] But such justice, essential as it may be for good morals, is not all that the Pythagorean ideal of justice implies. To the adherents of this dogma, justice was the social virtue par excellence. As Aristoxenus reports,[114] they believed that "in any relation with others" some kind of justice is involved. "In all intercourse" it is possible to take "a well-timed and an ill-timed attitude." In order to do what is proper, one must differentiate according to circumstances. Speech and actions necessarily vary depending on the particular situation and the persons concerned. From the right decision result timeliness, appropriateness, and fitness of behavior, and it is justice that reveals itself in good manners.[115] Interpreted in the light of Pythagorean teaching, then, the recommendation of justice epitomizes all duties of the physician towards his patient in the contacts of daily life, all he should do or say in the course of his practice; it gives the rules of medical deportment in a nutshell.[116]

Last but not least: the promise of silence. The physician accepts

[113] Cf. above, p. 33.

[114] 58 D 5, p. 470, 1 ff. [Diels-Kranz]: ἐπεὶ δὲ καὶ ἐν τῇ πρὸς ἕτερον χρείᾳ ἔστι τις δικαιοσύνη, καὶ ταύτης τοιοῦτόν τινα τρόπον λέγεται ὑπὸ τῶν Πυθαγορείων παραδίδοσθαι. εἶναι γὰρ κατὰ τὰς ὁμιλίας τὸν μὲν εὔκαιρον, τὸν δὲ ἄκαιρον, . . . ἔστι γάρ τι ὁμιλίας εἶδος, ὃ φαίνεται νεωτέρῳ μὲν πρὸς νεώτερον οὐκ ἄκαιρον εἶναι, πρὸς δὲ τὸν πρεσβύτερον ἄκαιρον. . . . τὸν αὐτὸν δ' εἶναι λόγον καὶ περὶ τῶν ἄλλων παθῶν τε καὶ πράξεων καὶ διαθέσεων καὶ ὁμιλιῶν καὶ ἐντεύξεων. . . . ἀκόλουθα δὲ εἶναι καὶ σχεδὸν τοιαῦτα, οἷα συμπαρέπεσθαι τῇ τοῦ καιροῦ φύσει τήν τε ὀνομαζομένην ὥραν καὶ τὸ πρέπον καὶ τὸ ἁρμόττον, καὶ εἴ τι ἄλλο τυγχάνει τούτοις ὁμοιογενὲς ὄν.

[115] Such a concept of justice seems entirely different from what Greek philosophers in general understand by justice. Aristotle, N.E., 1126 b 36 ff., for instance discusses under temperance that which the Pythagoreans call justice. On the other hand, the Pythagorean definition of justice in part overlaps with the common one in so far as the law also touches upon conduct, cf. Aristotle, N.E., V, ch. 1, and above, p. 35. In Aristoxenus' representation Pythagorean ethics often approximates the tenets of popular reflection, cf. Zeller, op. cit., I, 1, p. 460, and above, p. 30, n. 92.

[116] Deichgräber, who was the first to emphasize the importance which the concept of justice has in the Oath (op. cit., pp. 37; 41 ff.), goes so far as to say that the Oath embodies the ideal of the just physician (cf. above, p. 4, n. 5). This in my opinion is an exaggeration because the Oath combines the ideal of justice with that of forbearance (cf. above, p. 34); moreover, holiness and purity are also insisted upon (cf. above, p. 18). Justice then, important as it is, is not the only standard which is here applied to human actions. Cf. also below, p. 38, n. 123.

the obligation to keep to himself all that he sees or hears during the treatment; he also swears not to divulge whatever comes to his knowledge outside of his medical activity in the life of men.[117] The latter phrase in particular has always seemed strange. It is so far-reaching in scope that it can hardly be explained by professional considerations alone.[118] To be sure, other medical writings also advise the physician to be reticent. The motive in doing so is the concern for the physician's renommée which might suffer if he is a prattler.[119] But the Oath demands silence in regard to that "which on no account one must spread abroad." It insists on secrecy not as a precaution but as a duty.[120] In the same way silence about things which are not to be communicated to others was considered a moral obligation by the Pythagoreans. They did not tell everything to everybody. They did not indiscriminately impart their knowledge to others. They expected the scientist to be reticent and ready to listen.[121] They observed silence even in daily life. That they were taciturn beyond all other men no less than the fact that they were

---

[117] Cf. above, p. 2, 22-24.

[118] Cf. Jones, op. cit., p. 50.

[119] Cf. Hippocrates, Περὶ ἰητροῦ, C. M. G., I, 1, p. 20, 9: τὰ δὲ περὶ τὴν ψυχὴν σώφρονα, μὴ μόνον τῷ σιγᾶν . . . μέγιστα γὰρ ἔχει πρὸς δόξαν ἀγαθά. Deichgräber, op. cit., p. 37, refers to this passage; he himself admits that the statement serves merely utilitarian purposes.

[120] Incidentally, Körner, op. cit., p. 6, translates ἃ μὴ χρή ποτε ἐκλαλέεσθαι ἔξω by "wenn es nicht in die Öffentlichkeit gebracht werden muss," and in his interpretation, ibid., p. 17, states that this clause means that the physician should keep to himself everything except that which it is his duty to bring to public attention. In other words, Körner finds in the Oath a distinction between that which the physician owes to his patient and that which he owes to the community. Apart from the fact that the physician's obligations towards the state are nowhere mentioned in the document, such an interpretation is not warranted by the words. ἔξω is not "Öffentlichkeit" but simply "outside." Moreover, the text gives no indication as to what the physician should say, but only as to what he should keep to himself. Cf. also next note.

[121] Cf. Diogenes Laertius, VIII, 15 (Aristoxenus): μὴ εἶναι πρὸς πάντας πάντα ῥητά. Cf. 58 D 1, p. 467, 4 [Diels-Kranz]: σιωπηλοὺς δὲ εἶναι καὶ ἀκουστικοὺς . . . (from Aristoxenus after introductory remarks about the sciences accepted by the Pythagoreans [music, medicine, mantics]); cf. also below, pp. 46 f., concerning the transmission of knowledge in the Pythagorean school. Later, the ability to be reticent, in Pythagorean education, was considered the strongest proof of self-continence, the sign by which to distinguish good from bad pupils. Compare ἃ μὴ χρή in the Oath with Iamblichus, De Vita Pythagorica, 71: καὶ τὴν σιωπὴν καὶ τὴν λαλιὰν παρὰ τὸ δέον (from Apollonius [?]; cf. Rohde, op. cit., p. 137).

frugal in their habits made them the object of ridicule in ancient comedy.[122] Certainly if the doctor who promises not to talk about anything that he may see or hear is to be placed in any philosophical school, it must be the Pythagorean.

To sum up the results of the analysis of the ethical code: the provisions concerning the application of poison and of abortive remedies, in their inflexibility, intimated that the second part of the Oath is influenced by Pythagorean ideas. The interpretation of the other medical and ethical stipulations showed that they, too, are tinged by Pythagorean theories.[123] All statements can be understood only, or at any rate they can be understood best, as adaptations of Pythagorean teaching to the specific task of the physician. Even from a formal point of view, these rules are reminiscent of Pythagoreanism: just as in the Oath the doctor is told what to do and what not to do, so the Pythagorean oral instruction indicated what to do and what not to do.[124] Far from being the expression of the common Greek attitude towards medicine or of the natural duties of the physician, the ethical code rather reflects opinions which were peculiarly those of a small and isolated group.

[122] Cf. the fragment from Alexis, p. 479, 36 [Diels-Kranz]; cf. also, *ibid.*, p. 466, 20: γλώσσης πρὸ τῶν ἄλλων κράτει θεοῖς ἑπόμενος (old *Symbolon*), and *ibid.*, p. 97, 33 (Isocrates, *Busiris*, 29); in general cf. Zeller, *op. cit.*, III, 2, p. 80, n. 1. I need hardly refer to the proverbial *Silentium Pythagoricum.*

[123] Deichgräber, taking Apollo as the symbol of purity and justice, has characterized the morality advocated in the *Oath* as Apolline ethics, but this term as he uses it, is an invention *ad hoc* (*op. cit.*, p. 42: . . . "wenn man so will, die Idee des apollinischen Arztes"). To be sure, the Delphic religion promoted a certain ethical attitude, but the little that is known about it concerns men's relation to God and Fate rather than to his fellow men, cf. E. Howald, *Ethik des Altertums, Handbuch der Philosophie*, 1926, p. 11. An ethics as it is found in the Hippocratic *Oath* was a historical reality only in Pythagoreanism. That in some respects this philosophical system itself was influenced by Delphic concepts is possible; the ancients thought so themselves, cf. Diogenes Laertius, VIII, 8 (Aristoxenus). But such an agreement between Delphi and Pythagorean philosophy does not cover all those detailed injunctions in which the *Oath* coincides with the Pythagorean system.

[124] Cf. p. 464, 4 [Diels-Kranz]: Ἀκούσματα . . . τρία εἴδη . . . τὰ δὲ τί δεῖ πράττειν ἢ μὴ πράττειν. Deichgräber, *op. cit.*, p. 41, contends that the *Oath* "nur negative Bestimmungen enthält." Although the negative formulations are more numerous in the *Oath*, one cannot overlook the most emphatic positive statements concerning the physician's purity and holiness (cf. above, p. 2, 15-16), and concerning his promise to bring help to his patient (cf. above, p. 2, 12; 19).

II

THE COVENANT

The ethical code by the acceptance of which the physician gives a higher sanction to his practical endeavor is preceded by a solemn agreement concerning medical education. The pupil promises to regard his teacher as equal to his parents, to share his life with him, to support him with money if he should be in need of it. Next he vows to hold his teacher's children as equals to his brothers and to teach them the art without fee and covenant if they should wish to learn it. Finally he takes upon himself the obligation to impart precepts, oral instruction and all the other learning to his own sons, to those of his teacher and to pupils who have signed the covenant and have taken an oath according to the medical law, to all these, but to no one else.[1]

Whatever the precise purport of the single terms and phrases used in this covenant, so much is immediately clear in regard to its general meaning and is commonly admitted: the teacher here is made the adopted father of the pupil, the teacher's family becomes the pupil's adopted family. In other words, the covenant establishes between teacher and pupil the closest and most sacred relationship that can be imagined between men, and it does so for no other apparent reason than that the pupil is being instructed in the art.

In explaining this stipulation modern interpreters usually allege that in Greece, in early centuries, medicine like all the other arts was passed on from father to son in closed family guilds. When at a certain time these organizations began to receive outsiders into their midst, they are said to have demanded from them full participation in the responsibilities of the "real" children. Consequently those who wished to be admitted to all the privileges and rights of the family had to become its members through adoption. The Hippocratic covenant, then, it is claimed, is an engagement which was signed by newcomers joining one of the medical artisan families, and it was probably the family of the Asclepiads in which this formula held good.[2]

[1] Cf. above, p. 2, 5-11.
[2] Cf. e. g. Littré, op. cit., IV, pp. 611 ff.; I, pp. 341 ff.; Daremberg, op. cit., p. 2; for later proponents of this view, cf. Jones, op. cit., p. 44.

The evidence for such a theory, in my opinion, is insufficient. Galen is the only ancient author who asserts that the Asclepiads, after having been for generations the sole possessors of medicine, later shared their knowledge with people not belonging to their clan. And even he says that these outsiders were men whom the family esteemed " on account of their virtue "; he does not contend that they were made members of the family or forced to accept any obligations.[3] It is hardly by chance, therefore, that Galen himself does not refer to the Hippocratic Oath as bearing out the truth of his story. In any case, his words cannot be adduced as corroborative proof for the assumptions of modern scholars. Nor does it increase the strength of the modern argument if Galen's testimony is combined with that of Plato, according to whom " physicians taught their sons medicine and . . . Hippocrates taught outside pupils for a fee."[4] Though Plato says this, it still does not follow that the outsiders became the adopted children of their masters. On the contrary, who will believe that the young Athenian aristocrat Hippocrates of whom Plato speaks would have considered paying a fee to the great Hippocrates for instruction, had that meant that he should enter the family of the Coan physician![5]

If thus the usual interpretation of the Hippocratic covenant is unsupported by external testimony, it is equally unfounded as far as the wording of the text is concerned. For the covenant itself does not refer to a family guild of physicians. It speaks only of the pupil and the teacher, leaving open the question whether the latter is the son of a physician, the member of a clan of doctors, or not.[6] In view

[3] Cf. Galen, *Opera*, II, pp. 280 ff. K. The most important words are: . . . καὶ τοῖς ἔξω τοῦ γένους ἔδοξε καλὸν (!) εἶναι μεταδιδόναι τῆς τέχνης . . . ἤδη γὰρ τελέοις ἀνδράσιν, οὓς ἐτίμησαν ἀρετῆς ἕνεκα, ἐκοινώνουν τῆς τέχνης.

[4] Cf. Jones, *op. cit.*, p. 56; the Platonic passages referred to are *Laws*, IV, 720 b; *Protagoras*, 311 b. Substantially the same considerations are to be found in Littré, *op. cit.*, IV, pp. 611 ff., and in most authors who take the covenant as a document indicative of the state of family organizations.

[5] Cf. *Protagoras*, 311 b. Hirschberg, *op. cit.*, p. 28, seems the only one to admit that Plato does not give evidence for the *Oath*. For he emphasizes that in Plato's time the regulations found in the Hippocratic covenant—which he considers early—did no longer exist.

[6] As far as I know Jones has been the first to stress this fact. Cf. Jones, *Hippocrates*, I, p. 293: " Some scholars regard the *Oath* as the test required by the Asclepiad Guild. The document, however, does not contain a single word

of this fact it does not help to concede, as some scholars have done, that adoptions of outsiders into artisan families are hardly known from any other source, and yet to maintain that the Hippocratic covenant only confirms what must be presumed anyhow on the basis of generally valid laws of economic development. In all civilizations, it is stated, crafts were first restricted to family guilds; eventually these organizations became mere trade unions accessible to all; in a transitory period between these two stages the families adopted outsiders as "quasi-children." [7] I am not prepared to discuss the correctness of these so-called economic laws, nor do I wish to judge whether they are applicable to the Greek situation. The Hippocratic covenant at all events neither confirms such a theory, nor can it be explained by it; for there is no indication in the text that the document is concerned with family interests or family politics. [8]

Yet, if through the covenant the pupil is not received into a family guild, if he is made rather the adopted son of his teacher—was such a relationship common among the Greeks of any period? Some scholars answer this question in the affirmative. In the time preceding that of the Sophists, they say, the teacher generally was esteemed as the "spiritual father" of his pupil. [9] But this assertion

which supports this contention. It binds the student to his master and his master's family, not to a guild or corporation." Cf. also *The Doctor's Oath*, p. 56: "a private agreement between master and apprentice." Nevertheless Jones accepts the general view (*ibid.*, p. 44) that the covenant has something to do with the Asclepiad guild; but cf. also below, p. 47, n. 28.

[7] Cf. Deichgräber, *op. cit.*, pp. 32 ff. He says, p. 32: ". . . eine Idee, wie wir sie vielleicht im griechischen Vereinswesen hier und dort voraussetzen dürfen, aus antiken Nachrichten aber kaum kennen." As a matter of fact, even E. Ziebarth, *Das griechische Vereinswesen*, 1896, p. 96, to whom Deichgräber refers, apparently in explanation of his "vielleicht" and "kaum" (n. 18), knows of no other testimony than the Hippocratic *Oath*. Concerning Galen, II, p. 280, cf. above, p. 40. Plato, *Republic*, X, 599 c and *Fragmenta Historicorum Graecorum*, ed. G. Müller, II, 1848, p. 263, passages which Ziebarth quotes in addition, do not yield anything concerning the problem of adoption.

[8] I should mention that in consequence of the usual interpretation of the covenant different ethical standards have to be presupposed for the two sections of the *Oath* (cf. above, p. 4). To use the characterization of Deichgräber who has most strongly brought out this discrepancy (*op. cit.*, p. 38; p. 42): the first part shows a business point of view, whereas the second is determined by Apolline concepts of purity. Concerning this problem, cf. also above, p. 38, n. 123, and below, pp. 50 ff.

[9] Cf. E. Hoffmann, Kulturphilosophisches bei den Vorsokratikern, *Neue Jahr-*

can be made only if the Hippocratic covenant is taken as the basis
for speculations and generalizations which are not warranted by any
additional evidence. Granted that the covenant is determined by a
concept of spiritual kinship between teacher and pupil, it is nowhere
attested that the same idea prevailed in all schools and guilds of the
pre-classical era, or in any of them for that matter.[10] Surely, it is
not permissible to conclude from the covenant that the lack of such
evidence in regard to other than medical teaching in the 6th and
early 5th centuries is merely fortuitous. For it is uncertain when
the Hippocratic Oath was composed, and the document which itself
needs explanation and identification cannot possibly serve as the
starting point for theorizing about otherwise unknown circumstances.[11] There is no reason, then, to assume that the adoption of
the pupil by the teacher was a common characteristic of archaic
education. Nor is such a practice known to have been customary in
ancient scientific or practical training at any other time.[12]

bücher f. Wissenschaft u. Jugendbildung, V, 1929, pp. 19-20. This article, in spite
of its importance, is strangely neglected in the literature on the Oath.

[10] Hoffmann, loc. cit., says: "Über andere als ärztliche Schulen haben wir aus
jener Zeit leider nur Legenden, aber diese Legenden sagen uns ganz Ähnliches.
In dem Bunde der Pythagoreer z. B. war die Treue unter den Schülern des
Meisters wie die Treue zwischen Brüdern: Damon und Phintias. Die geistigen
Söhne des Meisters sind eben Brüder." Hoffmann himself, then, admits that these
stories portray situations only distantly related to those of the Oath, for he speaks
only of "similarity." Note, moreover, that the legend of Damon and Phintias to
which alone Hoffmann refers in proof of his statement concerns events taking
place in the 4th century B. C., in the time of Dionysius of Syracuse; cf. p. 472,
1 ff. [Diels-Kranz]. In view of the uncertainty in regard to the history of the old
Pythagorean school (cf. above, pp. 18 f.), it is impossible simply to reconstruct
conditions of the 6th century on the evidence of the 4th century. Finally, even if
the old Pythagorean society was a fraternity and was based on a spiritual kinship
with the master, Pythagoras would not necessarily be the direct teacher of his
pupils as is the master of the covenant; he would be the teacher and father
of all Pythagoreans, even of those who lived long after him, because he was the
founder of the school. In how far the covenant is determined also by a concept of
spiritual kinship between teacher and pupil will be discussed below, p. 57, n. 10.

[11] For the divergent assumptions concerning the date of the Oath, cf. below,
pp. 55 ff. Hoffmann's thesis which presupposes the pre-Sophistic origin of the Oath
without adducing any proof can be characterized only as ignotum per ignotius.

[12] S. Nittis, The Authorship and Probable Date of the Hippocratic Oath, Bulletin
of the History of Medicine, VIII, 1940, pp. 1012 ff., who takes the covenant as the
statute of a medical fraternity around 420 B. C., comparable to that of other

There is one particular historical setting, however, one particular province of Greek pedagogics where a counterpart of the Hippocratic covenant can be found: the Pythagoreans of the 4th century apparently were wont to honor those by whom they had been instructed as their fathers by adoption. So Epaminondas is said to have done; and in Epaminondas' time it was told of Pythagoras himself that he had revered his teacher as a son reveres his father.[13] If the Hippocratic covenant is viewed against the background of such testimony, the specific form in which the pupil is here bound to his teacher is no longer an unexplainable and isolated phenomenon. Compared with Pythagorean concepts of teaching and learning as they were evolved in the 4th century B. C., the vow of the medical student assumes definite historical meaning.[14]

This result seems to imply that the covenant as a whole must be influenced by Pythagorean philosophy. The agreement between the Hippocratic treatise and the Pythagorean reports concerns so unusual a circumstance that they are most unlikely to be independent of each other. Nor is it probable that the Pythagoreans derived their pattern of instruction from a medical manifesto that in the range of medical education and indeed of general education is without parallel.[15] Nevertheless one should hesitate to claim Pythagorean origin for the covenant by reason of one feature only, even if it be the main feature of this document.[16] But as matters stand, all the other demands enjoined upon the pupil may likewise be explained

fraternal societies of this time and later centuries, has not succeeded in finding one instance where in such organizations the pupil was adopted by the teacher.

[13] Cf. Diodorus, X, 11, 2: καὶ πατὴρ αὐτοῦ (sc. of Epaminondas) θετὸς ἐγένετο δι' εὔνοιαν (sc. his teacher Lysis); cf. Plutarch, De Genio Socratis, ch. 13, 583 C: . . . πατὴρ . . . ἐπιγραφείς. That the expression does not indicate a particular attachment of Epaminondas to Lysis is evident from what Diodorus, X, 3, 4, says about Pythagoras' relation to his teacher, Pherecydes: ὡσανεί τις υἱὸς πατέρα (Aristoxenus, cf. p. 44, 34 [Diels-Kranz]). Aristoxenus, too, relates of Epaminondas, p. 104, 3 [Diels-Kranz]: καὶ πατέρα τὸν Λῦσιν ἐκάλεσεν (for the source of this passage, cf. ibid., p. 103, n. 13). In these passages which Hoffmann apparently overlooked the father-son relation is expressly attested, and it is supposed to exist between the pupil and his teacher, just as in the Hippocratic Oath.

[14] Hoffmann, then, was fundamentally right in his suggestion that the Hippocratic Oath and Pythagorean doctrine are related, though the details of his argument are erroneous.

[15] Cf. above, p. 42.   [16] Cf. above, p. 39.

only in connection with Pythagorean views and customs, or at least they are compatible with them.

To take those duties first which the pupil acknowledges in regard to his mentor: he is asked to share his life with his teacher and to support him with money if need be.[17] This statement usually is considered an extravagant exaggeration that cannot be taken at its face value. Or, to avoid the stumbling block of excessive and improbable magnanimity, the words are said really to signify that the pupil should share with his master his livelihood, not his life, and if need be support him with money. Such an interpretation, however, itself falls prey to the objection that it gives to certain terms an unusual sense and makes the two stipulations of which the sentence consists meaningless repetitions.[18] In the light of what is known about the Pythagoreans the words chosen ring true. That the Pythagorean pupil shared his money with his teacher if necessary, one may readily believe. To support his father was the son's duty, even according to common law. This obligation was the more binding for the Pythagorean who was taught to honor his parents above all others.[19] But the Pythagorean also came to his teacher's assistance in all the vicissitudes of life, wherever and whenever he was needed: he tended

[17] Cf. above, p. 2, 5-6.

[18] For the former view, cf. e. g. Jones, *Hippocrates*, I, p. 292: "Indeed, such clauses could never be enforced; if they could have been, and if a physician had one or two rich pupils, his financial position would have been enviable." *Ibid.*, p. 295: "These (*sc.* clauses) might well contain promises to the teacher couched in extravagant language if taken literally, but which were intended to be interpreted in the spirit rather than in the letter." For the reinterpretation of the text, cf. e. g. Jones, *The Doctor's Oath*, p. 9: "To make him partner in my livelihood, and when he is in need of money to share mine with him"; Deichgräber, *op. cit.*, p. 31: "Mit ihm den Unterhalt zu teilen und ihn mitzuversorgen, falls er Not leidet." If pupil and teacher share their livelihood, how can the one be in need without the other being in need also? Or how could the one support the other in such a case? For βίος in the sense in which I have translated it, cf. the *Oath* itself, above, p. 2, 16; 26. Incidentally, Deichgräber, *op. cit.*, n. 7, rightly rejects as unwarranted Ziebarth's interpretation, *op. cit.*, p. 97, according to which the second part of the sentence is supposed to mean that if need be the pupil has to pay the teacher's debts.

[19] For the Pythagorean insistence on the reverence to be paid to parents, cf. Diogenes Laertius, VIII, 23: ἀνθρώπων δὲ μάλιστα τοὺς γονέας (*sc.* τιμᾶν); cf. p. 469, 12 ff. [Diels-Kranz] (Aristoxenus). In addition, one must remember that, according to Pythagorean doctrine, even friends shared everything, if one of them had lost his property, cf. below, p. 46, n. 25.

him in illness; he procured burial for him. All this is admiringly reported of Pythagoras himself.[20] The Pythagorean pupil was indeed supposed to share his life with his master, as the son does with his father. He did much more than advance money to him in case of an emergency.[21]

Next, the Hippocratic covenant admonishes the pupil to regard his teacher's offspring as his brothers, and without fee and covenant to teach them his art if they wish to learn it.[22] That the teacher's children should be the pupil's brothers naturally follows from the fact that the disciple acknowledges his master as his father. Thus the teacher's sons and his pupils become one flesh and blood.[23] But the preference shown for the interest of the members of the family, the unselfishness commended in the relationship to them, the confi-

[20] Cf. Diodorus, X, 3, 4, and above, p. 43, n. 13. The same story is told by Iamblichus, De Vita Pythagorica, 183-84, who concludes with the following words: οὕτω περὶ πολλοῦ τὴν περὶ τὸν διδάσκαλον ἐποιεῖτο σπουδήν. This statement is perhaps taken from Nicomachus, cf. Rohde, op. cit., p. 159, but the story itself is older, as is clear from Diodorus and also from Aristoxenus, cf. above, p. 43, n. 13. For the Pythagorean emphasis on the importance of an appropriate burial, cf. Plutarch, De Genio Socratis, 585 E.

[21] The importance which such a life companionship had for the Pythagoreans in general is evident also from the name later given to them: κοινόβιοι, Iamblichus, De Vita Pythagorica, 29; cf. also the term συμβίωσις as characteristic of the relationship between the brothers, ibid., 81.

[22] Cf. above, p. 2, 7-8. Concerning the exact meaning of the term "covenant," συγγραφή, cf. below, p. 47, n. 29. Deichgräber, op. cit., n. 9, is certainly right in rejecting the interpretation "Schuldschein" as opposed to "barer Lohn" (μισθός) proposed by Th. Meyer-Steineg–W. Schonack, Hippokrates, Über Aufgaben u. Pflichten d. Arztes, Kleine Texte, 1913, nr. 120. Such a meaning of the word is not attested.

[23] Note that the pupil is asked to consider his teacher's children (γένος τὸ ἐξ αὐτοῦ) as his "male brothers" (ἀδελφοὶ ἄρρενες). Jones, op. cit., p. 9, translates "brothers"; he thinks that the word ἄρρενες is "quite otiose" (ibid., p. 43, n. 1). Deichgräber, op. cit., p. 31, translates "männliche Geschwister." Earlier interpretations are collected and rejected by Daremberg, op. cit., p. 6, n. 3. Daremberg himself translates "propres frères," ibid., p. 5. Yet in Greek law the rights of kin differ as to male and female lineage, the former preceding the latter; cf. W. Erdmann, Die Ehe im alten Griechenland, 1934, pp. 117 ff.; pp. 125-6. ἀδελφοὶ ἄρρενες therefore probably means "brothers of male lineage" (for ἄρρενες in this sense, cf. e. g. Isaeus, VII, 20). Thus the relationship between adopted and real children is made as close as possible. Note that in Carmen Aureum, 1. 4 (quoted below, p. 46, n. 25) the ἄγχιστ' ἐγγεγαῶτες are mentioned after the parents. They constitute the so-called ἀγχιστεία which is contrasted with the relatives of female lineage even in the late laws of Charondas, cf. Diodorus, XII, 15, 2, and Erdmann, op. cit., p. 134, n. 62.

dence put in their reliability without any insistence on formal guarantees — all these features are characteristic of Pythagorean ethics.[24] The Pythagoreans were admonished to turn to their brothers first, and to make friends with them before all others outside the family. Moreover, all Pythagoreans considered themselves brothers and were believed, like brothers, to have divided their earthly goods among themselves. Their unquestioned belief in their brothers' trustworthiness did not falter even in the face of death.[25] Under these circumstances, how could the Pythagorean do other than teach his adopted brothers without fee the knowledge which he had acquired? What assurances could he expect or ask of them before he instructed them in the art that he had learned from their father?

Finally, the fact that in the Hippocratic covenant teaching is divided into precepts, oral instruction and the other learning,[26] is best understood as a Pythagorean classification. The precepts of Pythagoras, handed down from one generation to the other, were greatly renowned throughout the centuries. "Oral instruction" and "learning" were the two categories under which Aristoxenus listed all that was "taught and said" in Pythagorean circles, and all that the members of the school tried "to learn and remember."[27]

[24] That the form of a " Hausgemeinschaft " which is envisaged in the Hippocratic covenant is also typically Pythagorean will be shown below, pp. 57 f.

[25] For the seeking of their brothers' friendship, cf. Sotion, *Fragmenta Philosophorum Graecorum*, II, p. 47 [Mullach]: οἱ ἀδελφοὺς παρέντες καὶ ἄλλους φίλους ζητοῦντες παραπλήσιοι τοῖς τὴν ἑαυτῶν γῆν ἐῶσι, τὴν δὲ ἀλλοτρίαν γεωργοῦσιν (Sotion is a Neo-Pythagorean of the 1st century A. D.; cf. F. Susemihl, *Geschichte der Griechischen Literatur*, II, 1892, p. 332, n. 459); cf. *Carmen Aureum*, l. 4: σούς τε γονεῖς τίμα, τούς τ᾽ ἄγχιστ᾽ ἐγγεγαῶτας; but the statements seem to echo old tradition, cf. the insistence on family relations, Diogenes Laertius, VIII, 23, quoted above, p. 44, n. 19; cf. also below, pp. 57 f. For the Pythagorean communism, cf. Diodorus, X, 3, 5 : ὅτι ἐπειδάν τινες τῶν συνήθων ἐκ τῆς οὐσίας ἐκπέσοιεν, διῃροῦντο τὰ χρήματα αὐτῶν ὡς πρὸς ἀδελφούς. Cf. also Aristoxenus, p. 472, 16 ff. [Diels-Kranz], and Diogenes Laertius, VIII, 10; Gellius, *Noctes Atticae*, I, 9, 12. For the Pythagorean willingness to respond unhesitatingly to every demand made by one of their brothers, cf. the famous story of Phintias and Damon, Aristoxenus, p. 472, 1 ff. [Diels-Kranz]. Note especially ἡ προσποίητος πίστις (*ibid.*, p. 472, 7), and ἔφη οὖν ὁ Διονύσιος θαυμάσαι τε καὶ ἐρωτῆσαι, εἰ ἔστιν ὁ ἄνθρωπος οὗτος, ὅστις ὑπομενεῖ θανάτου γενέσθαι ἐγγυητής (*ibid.*, p. 472, 19).

[26] Cf. above, p. 2, 8-11.

[27] The terms used in the covenant are: παραγγελίη, ἀκρόησις, ἡ λοιπὴ μάθησις. For the first of these, cf. Aristoxenus, p. 477, 13 [Diels-Kranz] : παραγγέλματα (sc. of Pythagoras). For the second and third, cf. μαθήσεις καὶ ἀκροάσεις, Aristoxenus,

That knowledge, according to the covenant, is to be imparted to a closed circle of selected people alone, most assuredly is in agreement with those principles on which the transmission of Pythagorean doctrine was based. The Pythagoreans differed from all other philosophical sects in that they did not divulge their teaching to everybody.[28] They carefully examined those who wished to join them. It is attested even that they exacted an oath from the pupil who was to be admitted, just as the Hippocratic treatise speaks of outsiders who sign the covenant and take an oath before they are allowed to participate in the course of studies.[29]

To sum up: not only the main feature of the covenant, the father-

ibid., p. 467, 18. The exact meaning of these words is difficult to ascertain. Παραγγέλματα are maxims, perhaps similar to what in other reports are called ἀκούσματα, short practical rules without rational explanation, cf. p. 463, 33 [Diels-Kranz]; ἀκροάσεις probably are lectures; and μάθησις should comprise all other studies, whether theoretical or practical. Similarly the terms may also be used in the Hippocratic covenant. Cf. also next note. Whatever the correct explanation may be, one need not agree with Jones' statement, *op. cit.*, p. 43, n. 1: " . . . I feel sure that all scholars will consider the division of instruction into παραγγελίη, ἀκρόησις, and ἡ λοιπή μάθησις curious and unusual."

[28] Cf. Diogenes Laertius, VIII, 15, quoted above, p. 37, n. 121 (Aristoxenus), and in general Zeller, *op. cit.*, I, 1, pp. 315 ff. On account of the restriction of teaching demanded in the covenant one cannot explain παραγγελίη, ἀκρόησις, μάθησις (cf. preceding note) by parallels taken from non-Pythagorean schools of philosophy, or from other Hippocratic writings (cf. *e. g.* Daremberg, *op. cit.*, p. 7, n. 5; Jones, *op. cit.*, p. 9, n. 2). For these schools were open to everybody, and ἀκρόησις in Ps. Hippocrates, Παραγγελίαι, ch. XII, means "lecture before a crowd," just as the Παραγγελίαι themselves with which Jones compares the παραγγελίη of the covenant (*op. cit.*, p. 9, n. 2) formed a published book available to every reader. Incidentally, Jones, *op. cit.*, p. 45, refers to the Pythagoreans who, he says, perhaps held meetings from which outsiders were excluded. But he does not make use of this parallel for the interpretation of the *Oath*.

[29] For the Pythagorean Oath. cf. below, pp. 53 f. The covenant refers to pupils who are συγγεγραμμένοι τε καὶ ὡρκισμένοι νόμῳ ἰητρικῷ; Jones, *op. cit.*, p. 9, translates: "who have signed the indenture and sworn obedience to the physician's Law." But Deichgräber's rendering, *op. cit.*, p. 31: "vertraglich verpflichtet und vereidigt nach ärztlichem Brauch" seems more correct. The ξυγγραφή referred to here obviously is the same from which the teacher's children are exempted, cf. above, p. 45; but it is hardly identical with the covenant which the *Oath* contains, cf. below, p. 49. Nittis, *op. cit.*, p. 1019, says that the phrase implies that "others (*sc.* those who were not sons of physicians) had to qualify by a test, enrollment in the society, which naturally meant meeting the financial obligations of the association, taking the *Oath* and the payment of tuition." Not only does the covenant not concern societies, but as far as I can see, ξυγγραφή never has the meaning given to it by Nittis.

son relationship between teacher and pupil, but also all the detailed stipulations concerning the duties of the pupil can be paralleled by doctrines peculiar to the followers of Pythagoras.[30] If related to Pythagoreanism, the specific formulas used in the covenant acquire meaning and definiteness. What otherwise appears exaggerated, or strange, or even fictitious, thus becomes the adequate expression of a real situation. Since the rules proposed show no affinity with any other Greek educational theory or practice, it seems permissible to claim that the Hippocratic covenant is inspired by Pythagorean doctrine.

[30] As far as I am aware, my interpretation has covered all the points mentioned in the covenant, except the payment of a teaching-fee by the outside student, a regulation to be inferred from the fact that fees are remitted to the children of the master (cf. above, p. 45). The evidence available does not indicate, whether the Pythagoreans took money for instruction. But even Hippocrates taught medicine for a fee (cf. Plato, *Protagoras*, 311 b), and many philosophers charged money for their courses.

III

THE UNITY OF THE DOCUMENT

Covenant and ethical code, the two parts of which the so-called Hippocratic Oath consists, in the preserved text form a unity. Without any marked transition the first section is followed by the second.[1] Is there any reason for believing that the two have not always belonged together?

It seems certain that the obligations laid down in the covenant and in the ethical code are assumed by the physician simultaneously, that is, at the moment of his entering the medical profession as a practitioner in his own right. The promise to help the teacher and the stipulation concerning the teaching to be given to others point to the fact that he who takes the Oath has become an independent craftsman.[2] In the same way the rules regarding the practitioner's behavior are best understandable if imposed upon the doctor who is now starting out on his career. For as long as the pupil is still under the supervision of his teacher, his actions of necessity are regulated by his master's orders. In short, covenant and ethical code are signed together, not by the beginner but rather by the student who has completed his course.[3]

---

[1] It should be noted, however, that the covenant is given in infinitives, whereas the code is given in the first person. That this difference in style is an indication of archaic speech Deichgräber, *op. cit.*, p. 30, n. 3, has assumed but has not proved; that it is indicative of an original independence of the two sections is quite possible. Perhaps the covenant originally was used in various fields of instruction and was only taken over into the medical manifesto; if that were so, it would be easier to understand why the covenant refers to "the art" instead of to medicine. This, no doubt, would be a better explanation of this strange fact than the one given by Jones, *op. cit.*, pp. 50-51, who says that the physician "here called his profession, with glorious arrogance, 'the art'." Incidentally, the juxtaposition of aorist and future tenses which Jones blames as incorrect, *op. cit.*, p. 7; p. 43, n. 1, is not an uncommon usage, cf. Kühner-Gerth, *Griechische Grammatik*, II, 1, § 389, p. 195 A 7, esp. p. 197 *finis*.

[2] Moreover, as Deichgräber has rightly pointed out, *op. cit.*, p. 32, the covenant mentions another oath, apparently sworn before instruction begins.

[3] Cf. Deichgräber, *op. cit.*, p. 32: ". . . der Schwörende, offenbar ein Schüler, der nach Abschluss der Ausbildung in die Praxis geht, ..." Jones, *op. cit.*, p. 44; pp. 56 ff., seems to be of the same opinion, but he characterizes the covenant as an agreement between pupil and teacher, while he calls the ethical code an

Moreover the two parts are a spiritual unity. For it is not true, contrary to what is sometimes claimed, that the covenant exhibits a realistic business attitude, whereas the ethical code is determined by a lofty and exalted standard of conduct.[4] The agreement concerning teaching and the rules of professional behavior both reflect the same idealistic outlook on human affairs, they are steeped in Pythagorean doctrine. The same can be said of the preamble and the peroration by which the document is introduced and concluded as one coherent formula.

In the invocation, Apollo the physician, Asclepius and his children, and all the gods and goddesses are made witnesses of the vow to be taken.[5] That all the divine powers are called upon is the usual form in which an ancient oath, at least an oath of some importance, is pronounced, for this makes the protestation all the more solemn.[6] That Apollo the physician and his son Asclepius are named in particular is quite appropriate for a medical oath. It is also in agreement with Pythagorean views that a member of the medical profession should invoke these deities. According to Aristoxenus, the art of selecting the right food and drink for the human regimen, in the belief of the Pythagoreans, had first been practiced by Apollo and Paeon, while later it was taken over by the physicians, the sons of Asclepius. The Pythagorean doctor, the healer of diseases by diet, then, must have revered precisely the gods whom the Oath addresses.[7]

---

obligation toward the society of physicians. There is no reason for such a distinction, cf. below, pp. 61-62. It is true, as O. Temkin suggests, that because in ancient medicine the apprentice assisted his master in his practice (cf. *e. g.* Ps. Hippocrates, *Prorrhetikon*, II, IX, p. 20 L.), the ethical rules might apply to the student. Cf. also C. Singer, *A Short History of Medicine*, 1928, p. 17. Yet for the reasons just given it seems more likely that the *Oath* was administered after the teaching had ended and the pupil became responsible for his own actions.

[4] Cf. Deichgräber, *op. cit.*, p. 34; p. 38. Deichgräber fails to explain how statements of so different an ethos should ever have become a unity. Jones, who also sharply distinguishes the two parts, seems not to find any difference in regard to the ethical standards though in his opinion the covenant is somewhat at variance with the code, cf. especially, *op. cit.*, p. 43.

[5] Cf. above, p. 2, 2-4.

[6] Cf. E. Ziebarth, *De iure iurando*, 1892, pp. 17 ff.; Deichgräber, *op. cit.*, n. 13.

[7] Cf. p. 475, 32 f. [Diels-Kranz] (quoted above, p. 24, n. 65). Apollo the physician, as the *Oath* has it, obviously is Apollo and Paeon of whom Aristoxenus speaks; the two were often merged into one deity of medicine; cf. H. Usener, *Götternamen*, 1896, pp. 153 ff. Note that contrary to Deichgräber, *op. cit.*, p. 42, Apollo here is

That Asclepius' divine children, Panaceia and Hygieia, are called upon in addition is not astounding. The names of all the members of the divine medical family come naturally to the mind of the believer in Apollo and Asclepius when he takes upon himself those obligations that will guide his future life as a physician.[8]

Having invoked the gods as witnesses and having bound himself to live in purity and holiness, justice and forbearance, he who swears asks that he may enjoy his life and art in fame if the vow is kept inviolate; if it is not carried out, the opposite shall befall him.[9] Does this peroration indicate that in his very heart the physician is motivated not by ethical standards but rather by the wish to attain success? Is it his reputation that he wants to see enhanced by all his actions and that he forswears in case of his failure to fulfil his obligations?[10] This can hardly be the meaning of the words in question. For it is not fame or a good name among his clients for which the juror prays, it is fame for all time among all men, it is immortal fame that is here implored or renounced.[11] Such a wish one cannot reasonably call aspiring to a good reputation in the interest of business, though a good reputation was of great practical

not necessarily the Delphic god, the god of purity. The Delphic Apollo renounces medicine in favor of his son Asclepius, cf. Wilamowitz, *Der Glaube der Hellenen*, II, 1932, p. 35. Nor is he commonly regarded as patron of the physicians (Deichgräber, *ibid.*); statements to this effect, such as Callimachus, *Hymnus in Apollinem*, II, 45-6, are very rare. But for the Pythagoreans who reformed medicine according to their concept of purity and who introduced music into medicine (cf. p. 467, 13-15 [Diels-Kranz]), the Delphic Apollo may indeed have been identical with the god of medicine.

[8] For Hygieia and Panaceia as daughters of Asclepius, cf. *e. g. Paean Erythraeus in Aesculapium*, ed. I. U. Powell, *Collectanea Alexandrina*, 1925, p. 136.

[9] Cf. above, p. 2, 25-27. That the prayer for divine blessing is coupled with an execration is typical for a solemn oath; cf. R. Hirzel, *Der Eid*, 1902, p. 138; cf. also H. Schöne, *Sokrates*, I, 1913, p. 127; Deichgräber, *op. cit.*, n. 14. It should also be emphasized that it is usual to invoke the gods at the beginning, while at the end only the consequences that will ensue in this world are mentioned; cf. Hirzel, *op. cit.*, p. 69.

[10] Cf. Deichgräber, *op. cit.*, pp. 35-36, who sees in the wish for fame the confirmation of his opinion that even here the utilitarian point of view is not set aside. The physician's regard for his reputation, he thinks, is only tempered by his concern for what is right, *ibid.*, p. 41.

[11] Cf. above, p. 2, 26-27: δοξαζομένῳ παρὰ πᾶσιν ἀνθρώποις ἐς τὸν ἀεὶ χρόνον. The expression is as tautological as the words of Plato, *Symposium*, 208 c: κλέος ἐς τὸν ἀεὶ χρόνον ἀθάνατον καταθέσθαι.

importance for the ancient doctor.[12] Rather is this prayer characteristic of the Greek love for glory, of the ancient belief in eternal fame on this earth as a stimulus to all good deeds. No less a man than Solon, in exactly the words of the Oath, asks for renown among all future generations in recompense for what he has done and written. In the same vein Plato acknowledges that the craving for undying fame is the real motive of all great achievements.[13]

That such an insistence on glory is in the opinion of the Greeks entirely compatible with an idealistic attitude can be proved by many instances. Even the earliest philosopher who upheld a philanthropic and moral belief against the philosophy of success saw in glory the righteous aim of human actions.[14] Nor did the Pythagoreans shun this goal. Aristoxenus reports that they were opposed only to such glory as consists in the approbation of the many, but thought it foolish to despise all fame.[15] It is for this reason that glory, though sometimes deprecated by the Pythagoreans and grouped together with the vices, in other instances is extolled as praiseworthy.[16] Most important: the Pythagoreans, too, were striving for that glory which

---

[12] I am the last to deny the significance which the physician's regard for reputation had in ancient medicine; cf. L. Edelstein, *Problemata*, IV, 1931, chap. III. But the attitude outlined in the *Oath* is enjoined in opposition to the realities and exigencies of daily life; here an attempt is made to better existing conditions, to remedy the rather deplorable state of affairs, cf. below, p. 59.

[13] Cf. Solon, I, 3-4: ὄλβον μοι πρὸς θεῶν μακάρων δότε καὶ πρὸς ἀπάντων/ ἀνθρώπων αἰεὶ δόξαν ἔχειν ἀγαθήν. Plato, *Symposium*, 208 c ff.; cf. also Pindar, *Isthmiae*, IV, 12; and in general J. Burkhardt, *Griechische Kulturgeschichte*, ed. J. Oeri, IV³, pp. 233 ff. (for the heroic time, *ibid.*, p. 17).

[14] I am thinking of the so-called *Anonymus Iamblichi*, 89 [Diels-Kranz]; cf. especially II, p. 402, 19-20 [Diels-Kranz]; cf. in general W. Capelle, *Die Griechische Philosophie*, II, 1, p. 24 (Göschen nr. 858) and also R. Roller, *Untersuchungen zum Anonymus Iamblichi*, Diss. Tübingen, 1931. Cf. below p. 53, n. 18.

[15] Cf. p. 473, 32 ff. [Diels-Kranz]: ἀνόητον μὲν εἶναι καὶ τὸ πάσῃ καὶ παντὸς δόξῃ προσέχειν . . . ἀνόητον δ' εἶναι καὶ πάσης ὑπολήψεώς τε καὶ δόξης καταφρονεῖν. (In the index of Kranz this passage is said to deal with δόξα in the sense of " opinion "; but δόξα παρὰ τῶν πολλῶν, lines 33-4, clearly is " fame "; note also the connection in which the passage is quoted by Iamblichus). A very similar statement is found in Iamblichus, *Protrepticus*, ch. 6, p. 40, 7 [Pistelli]; cf. also Iamblichus, *De Vita Pythagorica*, 72 (Apollonius), cf. Rohde, *op. cit.*, p. 137.

[16] Cf. such passages as p. 471, 23 [Diels-Kranz] (φιλοτιμία, ἐπιθυμία, ὀργή), or Iamblichus, *De Vita Pythagorica*, 69 (δόξα, πλοῦτος); cf. also *ibid.*, 188; 226. On the other hand, cf. *ibid.*, 223: . . . τὴν σωτηρίαν τῆς ἐννόμου δόξης, δι' ἣν αὐτός τε μόνα τὰ δοκοῦντα ἑαυτῷ ἔπραττε . . . .

makes a man's name live for all time to come. Pythagoras himself was said to have exhorted his pupils to philosophical endeavor by stating that "education stays with men unto death, and for some it brings immortal fame even after death."[17] No doubt, the Pythagoreans approved of the desire for fame. The physician who prays for glory does not violate the code of Pythagorean ethics.[18]

Yet one may object: even granted that the content of the invocation and the peroration seems to be Pythagorean, were the followers of Pythagoras allowed to take an oath, to swear in the names of the gods? Certainly some Pythagorean sources stipulate that one should not swear by the gods, but should rather make oneself the witness of one's own words.[19] Still this hardly means that the Pythagoreans intended to ban all oaths and all invocations of divine witnesses. No Greek could ever have gone that far.[20] It is true, "Pythagoras" tried to remedy the notorious Greek predilection for making oaths. Yet the aim of the Pythagoreans was the restriction, not the abolition of vows. As Diodorus expressly states, in the opinion of the school, an oath should be sworn only on rare occasions.[21] Even the

[17] Cf. Iamblichus, *De Vita Pythagorica*, 42: . . . τῆς δὲ παιδείας καθάπερ οἱ καλοὶ κἀγαθοὶ τῶν ἀνδρῶν μέχρι θανάτου παραμενούσης, ἐνίοις δὲ καὶ μετὰ τὴν τελευτὴν ἀθάνατον δόξαν περιποιούσης (from Timaeus through Apollonius [cf. Rohde, *op. cit.*, p. 134; P. Corssen, *Sokrates*, I, 1913, pp. 199 ff.]; "aus . . . Bruchstücken ächter Tradition" [Rohde, *ibid.*]).

[18] Burckhardt, *Griechische Kulturgeschichte*, IV, p. 166; *Vorträge*, p. 198, holds that Pythagoras was the only philosopher who opposed the Greek craving for glory. But Porphyry, *Vita Pythagorae*, 32: φιλοτιμίαν φεύγειν καὶ φιλοδοξίαν (from Diogenes), the only passage quoted by Burckhardt, must be interpreted in the light of the testimony of Aristoxenus referred to above, p. 52, n. 15. In addition it should be noted that the idealistic ethical system to which I have alluded (cf. above, p. 52, n. 14) is known only from Iamblichus who integrates these passages into his *Protrepticus* as the final incentive to the study of philosophy. The name of the author whom he follows is unknown (cf. II, p. 400, n. 1 [Diels-Kranz]). Could he have been a Pythagorean?

[19] Cf. Diogenes Laertius, VIII, 22: μηδ' ὀμνύναι θεούς· ἀσκεῖν γὰρ αὐτὸν δεῖν ἀξιόπιστον παρέχειν (from Androcydes, thus Corssen, *Rh. M.*, LXVII, 1912, p. 258).

[20] Cf. Hirzel, *op. cit.*, p. 112, who points out the difference between this attitude and that of the Jews and Christians.

[21] Diodorus, X, 9, 2: ὅτι Πυθαγόρας παρήγγελε τοῖς μανθάνουσι σπανίως μὲν ὀμνύναι, . . . ; cf. Hirzel, *op. cit.*, pp. 98 ff.; Burckhardt, *Griechische Kulturgeschichte*, III, p. 320. H. Diels, *Archiv f. Geschichte d. Philosophie*, III, 1890, p. 457, does not do justice to this divergence of the tradition. Diodorus' statement most probably goes back to Aristoxenus on whom he largely depends, cf. E.

late Pythagoreans, though they seem to have been stricter in this respect, did not renounce vows altogether. Just as the physician is supposed to take an oath when he settles down to practice, so those who intended to become members of the Pythagorean society took an oath of allegiance.[22]

At this point, I think, I can say without hesitation that the so-called Oath of Hippocrates is a document, uniformly conceived and thoroughly saturated with Pythagorean philosophy. In spirit and in letter, in form and content, it is a Pythagorean manifesto. The main features of the Oath are understandable only in connection with Pythagoreanism; all its details are in complete agreement with this system of thought. If only one or another characteristic had been uncovered, one might consider the coincidence fortuitous. Since the concord is complete, and since there is no counterinstance of any other influence, all indications point to the conclusion that the Oath is a Pythagorean document.

Schwartz, s. v. Diodorus, Pauly-Wissowa, V, p. 679, for it is in perfect agreement with Aristoxenus' compromising attitude, cf. above, p. 30, n. 92.

[22] For the Neo-Pythagoreans in general, cf. Zeller, op. cit., III, 2, p. 146 (I, 1, p. 462, n. 7), and again for the similarity of the Pythagorean attitude with that of the Essenians, ibid., III, 2, p. 284, n. 5; cf. also Hirzel, op. cit., pp. 99-100. Julian, VII, 236 D, probably in opposition to the Christians, says: . . . οὔτε τὸ ὅρκῳ χρῆσθαι προπετῶς τοῖς τῶν θεῶν ὀνόμασιν [sc. ἐπέτρεπεν]. Pétrequin, op. cit., p. 173, was the first to compare the Hippocratic Oath with Pythagorean fidelity to a vow.

IV

DATE AND PURPOSE OF THE OATH

The origin of the Hippocratic Oath having been established, it should now be possible to determine the time when the Oath was written and the purpose for which it was intended. What answers regarding these questions are to be deduced from the analysis of the document?

As for the date, it seems one must conclude that the Oath was not composed before the 4th century B. C. All the doctrines followed in the treatise are characteristic of Pythagoreanism as it was envisaged in the 4th century B. C.[1] It is most probable even that the Oath was outlined only in the second half or towards the end of the 4th century, for the greater part of the parallels adduced are taken from the works of pupils of Aristotle.

Yet is such an assumption not irreconcilable with certain external data? Aristophanes, it is said, in one of his comedies performed in 411 B. C. makes mention of the Hippocratic Oath.[2] Not even the ancient commentators dared to claim that the Hippocrates referred to here was the physician of Cos. Eager as they were to find allusions to great historical names wherever that was possible, and even where it was most unlikely, in the case in question they expressly stated that the Hippocrates whom Aristophanes names was an Athenian general.[3] Nor can one infer from linguistic considerations that the

[1] The only exceptions to this statement are the references to Sotion and to the *Carmen Aureum* (cf. above, p. 46, n. 25). I think it permissible to say that, the whole argument taken into consideration, these two instances do not invalidate the claim that the interpretation given rests on the testimony of 4th century authors.

[2] D. Triller in the 18th century seems to have been the originator of this claim. Littré first followed him, *op. cit.*, I, p. 31, but later rejected the theory, cf. *ibid.*, II, p. xlviii; IV, p. 610. Pétrequin, however, repeated Triller's argument, *op. cit.*, p. 172, n. 1, and it has again been brought forward by Jones, *op. cit.*, p. 40.

[3] Cf. Aristophanes, *Scholia in Thesmophoriazusas*, v. 273; in *Nubes*, v. 1001; and Daremberg, *op. cit.*, p. 1, n. 1. I must confess that I fail to discover any reference to an Oath of Hippocrates in the lines in question. Euripides swears by Aether, the abode of Zeus (272). The interlocutor asks why he does so instead of swearing τὴν Ἱπποκράτους ξυνοικίαν. This, Jones, *op. cit.*, p. 40, takes to mean: "by the community of Hippocrates." But ξυνοικία is a tenement house in which many families live, and it is apparently the joke of the whole statement that the inter-

55

Oath was written in the 5th century. Granted for the sake of argument that the great Hippocrates was the author of the Oath; that he was in Athens in the year 421 B. C.; that the words "covenant" and "law" in Athens between March and October, 421, were used interchangeably to cover the same meaning, just as they are supposedly used in the Oath—all this would have no bearing on the date of this document, for it is written in the Ionic, not in the Attic dialect.[4] There is, then, no reason for rejecting the date that seems to follow from the internal evidence on the basis of external data.[5]

On the other hand, one may argue: it is true, the Oath agrees with reports of 4th century writers on Pythagoreanism; yet these accounts, though they stem from the 4th century, must not necessarily describe the Pythagorean system as it was evolved or understood at that time; the passages may in part at least reflect older conditions or reproduce more ancient traditions; the composition of the Hippocratic Oath, therefore, could well fall into an earlier period. However, such reasoning is not probable. I shall not dwell on the fact that the Pythagorean system of the 5th or even of the 6th century is practically unknown, that whatever is reported about the old Pythagorean teaching as a whole is, if not the invention, at least the interpretation of authors of the 4th century.[6] Two of the main pro-

locutor does not understand why the oath should be made by the house of Zeus rather than by the house of Hippocrates. That by ξυνοικία "Aristophanes probably had in mind the opening words of Oath, with their comprehensive ξυνοικία of divinities" (Jones, *ibid.*), I cannot believe, the less so, since ξυνοικία is never used in the sense required by Jones' interpretation. It should also be noted that Athenaeus, III, 96 e-f, says that "the sons of Hippocrates were ridiculed in comedy for swinishness," a statement which certainly refers to the Aristophanes passages under discussion.

[4] Cf. Nittis, *Bulletin of the History of Medicine*, 1940, p. 1020. I am far from admitting that Nittis' statements concerning the terms νόμος and ξυγγραφή are convincing, but for the reason given above I see no need to go into the details of his theory. In regard to the external evidence, I should mention at least that the Hippocratic *Oath* in reality is first mentioned by Erotianus and by Scribonius Largus in the first century A. D. Erotianus' list of Hippocratic writings probably goes back to Hellenistic sources, but even so the *Oath* would not be attested before the 3rd century B. C. (cf. Deichgräber, *op. cit.*, n. 1).

[5] That the fifth century origin of the *Oath* cannot be proved by reference to general sociological laws has been shown above, p. 41.

[6] Cf. above, pp. 18 f.; in general Ueberweg-Praechter, *op. cit.*, pp. 67 ff.; cf. also *ibid.*, p. 66: "Im allgemeinen gilt, abgesehen von jener Lehre (*sc.* that of metem-

visions of the Oath are connected with theories that are attributed
either directly or indirectly to Philolaus, a contemporary of Plato.
This makes the turn of the 5th to the 4th century the *terminus post
quem* for the composition of the Oath.[7] Moreover, even if one or
another ethical precept ascribed to the Pythagoreans by Aristoxenus
and accepted in the Hippocratic Oath was held also by older Pythagoreans, the whole program of instruction envisaged in the Oath in
conformity with the Pythagorean model is characteristic f 4th century Pythagoreanism; for it presupposes the destruction of the
Pythagorean society in the last decades of the 5th century.[8] As Aristoxenus relates, it was after the uprising in Italy that Lysis went to
Thebes where he taught Epaminondas and was revered by him as
his adopted father. In a letter ascribed to him, Lysis protes's against
those who after the dissolution of the society made the Pythagorean
dogma available to everybody. Pythagoras himself, Lysis asserts,
had charged his daughter never to give his writings to those " outside
of the house." [9] Whether this letter is genuine or not, it must have
been for some such reasons that Lysis bound Epaminondas to himself
as his adopted son. This afforded the only solution which made it
possible to initiate outsiders into the Pythagorean doctrine, and yet
to keep it a secret, a " family secret," as is also the intention of the
Oath.[10] But such a relationship between teacher and pupil could be

psychosis), jedenfalls der Satz, dass wir nur von einer Philosophie der Pythagoreer,
nicht des Pythagoras sprechen können, wie dies in der Tat auch schon bei Aristoteles
geschieht." And these Pythagoreans, as far as their names are known, are Philolaus
and his contemporaries or successors, cf. *ibid.*, p. 61.

[7] For Philolaus and his relation to Plato, cf. *e. g.* Ueberweg-Praechter, *op. cit.*,
p. 65 (44 A 5 [Diels-Kranz]) ; cf. above, p. 15 and p. 17.

[8] For the time of the dissolution of the Pythagorean society through which the
members of the school were brought from Italy to Greece, cf. Zeller, *op. cit.*,
I, 1, pp. 332 ff ; Ueberweg-Praechter, *op. cit.*, p. 65; K. v. Fritz, Pythagorean
Politics in Southern Italy, 1940, p. 92.

[9] Cf. p. 104, 1 ff. [Diels-Kranz], and Diogenes Laertius, VIII, 42; Hercher,
Epistolographi Graeci, p. 603, 5. For the authenticity of the letter, cf. p. 421, 12 ff.
[Diels-Kranz]. The situation is viewed in the same manner by Aristoxenus, cf.
Diogenes Laertius, VIII, 15, and Timaeus, cf. *ibid.*, 54. Nicomachus also sum-
marizes the situation by asserting that the Pythagoreans restricted their teaching to
the members of their own families, cf. Iamblichus, *De Vita Pythagorica*, 253; 251;
Porphyry, *Vita Pythagorae*, 58. Nicomachus uses the same words ἔξω τῆς οἰκίας
which appear in the letter of Lysis.

[10] Cf. above, p. 45. The belief in a spiritual kinship between teacher and pupil (cf.

instituted only after the disappearance of the great fraternity that had existed before. Only at that moment did the transmission of the Pythagorean doctrine become the concern of the individual Pythagorean; in earlier times it had been promoted by the society itself. The Hippocratic Oath which calls the teacher the adopted father of the pupil can hardly have been composed, therefore, before the 4th century B. C.[11]

Nor is it likely that the document is of later origin. In the 4th century B. C. Pythagoreanism reached the peak of its importance. Its influence gradually began to wane from the beginning of the Hellenistic period. When in the 1st century B. C. the Pythagorean system was revived and again became a potent factor in philosophical speculation, it took on traits very different from those which are characteristic of the earlier dogma and the prescripts of the Oath.[12]

above, p. 41) may also have been influential in the founding of this system of education, for even in their ethical behavior the Pythagoreans were bidden to take toward each other the attitude of the good father toward his children, cf. p. 471, 24 [Diels-Kranz]; *ibid.*, 477, 15 (Aristoxenus), where again this fatherly love is compared with that of the benefactor; both must be free from envy. If men owe to nature their lives, but to education their knowledge of the right life (Diodorus, XII, 13, 3 [Charondas]; cf. Rohde, *op. cit.*, p. 168), the teacher can well be called the spiritual father of the pupil. But basically the insistence on an adoption of the pupil is determined by external factors, by the new situation in which the Pythagoreans found themselves in the 4th century B. C. In this connection it seems worth pointing out that in the Platonic *Phaedo* which is strongly influenced by Pythagorean concepts Socrates is once referred to as the father of his pupils (116 a), just as late Neo-Platonists for whom the Platonic and Pythagorean dogmas coincide, again speak of their teacher as their father and even of the teacher's teacher as their grandfather, cf. Marinus, *Vita Procli*, 29. For the importance of the father-son relation in later mystery cults, cf. R. Reitzenstein, *Die hellenistischen Mysterienreligionen*[3], 1927, p. 20 (cf. also first edition, 1910, p. 27).

[11] That the *Oath* cannot be traced to pre-Sophistic times for the reasons adduced by Hoffmann, has been shown above, p. 42. Meyer-Steineg–Schonack, *op. cit.*, p. 4, assume the date of the 6th century without even attempting to give a proof for their assertion; cf. also Deichgräber, *op. cit.*, n. 24.

[12] For the general development of Pythagoreanism, cf. Ueberweg-Prächter, *op. cit.*, p. 65; pp. 513 ff.; esp. p. 516. Even if the Pythagorean school was not entirely in eclipse in Hellenistic centuries, it certainly had lost its strong hold over the philosophical mind. Yet in the 4th century B. C. Pythagoreanism through Plato, Aristotle and their schools had become a subject of general interest for the educated. As the references in the Middle Comedy prove, the followers of Pythagoras were also figures familiar to everyone. The Neo-Pythagorean movement of the 1st century B. C. is influenced by mystic tendencies; the ascetic features are

Moreover, in Alexandria medical ethics was integrated into the teaching of the medical sects. Closely connected as these newly established schools were with philosophy, Pythagoreanism played no part in their teaching. A direct influence of Pythagorean philosophy on medicine, however, is not probable.[13]

Yet in the 4th century B. C. the Hippocratic Oath in every respect was a timely manifesto. In that period many individual attempts were made to improve medical conditions. Abuses, to be sure, had been criticized even before.[14] But it is in those Hippocratic treatises that were written in the second half of the 4th century or even later, that one finds the first outlines of a system of medical deontology. Moreover, these endeavors at reform were instigated by the reflection on ethical problems as it developed in the rising philosophical schools.[15] Thus a medical ethics devised in accordance with Pythagoreanism is well in agreement with the general trend of thought in that period. On the other hand, from the point of view of 4th century Pythagoreanism it was quite justifiable that those concepts which

overstressed; the practical interest in human affairs which the *Oath* presupposes, cf. below, p. 60, is almost entirely lacking. That is why I cannot believe that the *Oath* is in any way connected with this late teaching.

[13] It has sometimes been claimed that the Hippocratic *Oath* was written in Hellenistic times. The proof offered is the fact that medicine is here divided into dietetics, pharmacology and surgery, cf. Münzer, *Münchener medizinische Wochenschrift*, 1919, p. 309; cf. Körner, *op. cit.*, p. 7. That this division is not typical of Alexandrian medicine has been shown above, p. 20, n. 49. C. Singer, *From Magic to Science*, 1928, p. 18, goes so far as to say: " Despite the Ionic Greek dress in which this formula is known to us, there is evidence that it is of Imperial date, and of Roman rather than of Greek origin "; cf. the same, *A Short History of Medicine,* 1928, pp. 16 ff.: parts earlier than Hippocrates, the *Oath* as such very much later. Singer does not make explicit why he holds this belief.

[14] Cf. especially the surgical books of the *Corpus Hippocraticum* which are usually ascribed to the 5th century; cf. *e. g.* K. Deichgräber, Die Epidemien und das Corpus Hippocraticum, *Abh. Berl. Akad.*, 1933, nr. 3, p. 98. In general L. Edelstein, *Problemata*, IV, pp. 100 ff.

[15] I am referring to the books *Decorum, Physician* and *Precepts*. For their late date and for the Epicurean or Stoic influence on them, cf. Jones in his introduction to these treatises, Loeb vols. I and II; cf. also the chapter " Ancient medical etiquette," *ibid.*, II, pp. xxxiii ff. The Ps. Hippocratic *Law,* another book of this type, has been connected with the Democritean school by Wilamowitz, *Hermes,* LIV, 1919, pp. 46 ff.; cf. however, F. Müller, *Hermes*, LXXV, 1940, pp. 39 ff., who dates the treatise in the 5th century. I was unable to secure this article which is abstracted in *Classical Weekly,* XXXVI, 1942, p. 84.

underlay philosophical instruction were applied also to the teaching of the healing art, and that Pythagorean ethics was infused into the practice of medicine. The school ranked medicine together with music and mantic as the supreme sciences. Medical skill, to its members, was the greatest wisdom attainable by men.[16] The standards of medical education, therefore, could not be set too high. Moreover, the Pythagoreans thought that "love for what is truly noble" manifests itself in practical pursuits and in the sciences— for here the love for good habits and the devotion to them become apparent—and consequently they called the fair and dignified sciences "full of love for the noble." To imbue medicine with the spirit of Pythagorean holiness and purity was a task enjoined by the Pythagorean dogma itself.[17]

It stands to reason, then, that it was in the 4th century B. C. that Pythagorean philosophy led to the formulation of the Hippocratic Oath. Does this imply that the document must have been outlined by a philosopher rather than by a physician? Not at all. The Hippocratic Oath is a program of medical ethics, and there is no reason to question that it was composed by a doctor. But ancient physicians often belonged to philosophical schools or studied with philosophers. The Pythagorean teaching aroused considerable interest among the physicians of the 4th century.[18] It is quite possible that a physician,

[16] Cf. 58 D 1, p. 467, 3 [Diels-Kranz]: τῶν δ' ἐπιστημῶν οὐχ ἥκιστά φασιν τοὺς Πυθαγορείους τιμᾶν μουσικήν τε καὶ ἰατρικὴν καὶ μαντικήν (Aristoxenus); cf. ibid., p. 464, 9: τί σοφώτατον τῶν παρ' ἡμῖν; ἰατρική (old Ἄκουσμα).

[17] Cf. p. 478, 17 ff. [Diels-Kranz]: τὴν ἀληθῆ φιλοκαλίαν ἐν τοῖς ἐπιτηδεύμασι καὶ ἐν ταῖς ἐπιστήμαις ἔλεγεν εἶναι· . . . ὡσαύτως δὲ καὶ τῶν ἐπιστημῶν τε καὶ ἐμπειριῶν τὰς καλὰς καὶ εὐσχήμονας ἀληθῶς εἶναι φιλοκάλους . . . (Aristoxenus). What men gain in the usual pursuits of life only is λάφυρά που τῆς ἀληθινῆς . . . φιλοκαλίας. The term φιλοκαλία itself seems to be preeminently a Peripatetic concept, cf. N. E., 1125 b 12; 1179 b 9; cf. also E. E., 1250 b 34; 1251 b 36. It almost approaches the meaning of "love of honor," cf. Xenophon, Symposium, IV, 15. Zeller's interpretation of the fragment ("Die Wissenschaft . . . kann nur da gedeihen, wo sie mit Lust und Liebe betrieben wird," op. cit., I, 1, p. 462) does not do justice to the words.

[18] Thus Philolaus is mentioned in Meno's history of medicine, 44 A 27 [Diels-Kranz]. Androcydes, a physician, wrote on Pythagorean symbols, cf. C. Hölk, De acusmatis sive symbolis Pythagoricis, Diss. Kiel, 1894, pp. 40 ff.; Corssen, Rh. M., LXVII, 1912, pp. 240 ff. Another Pythagorean physician of that time (Phaon) is perhaps referred to in a fragment preserved from the Middle Comedy, p. 479, 26 [Diels-Kranz].

strongly impressed by what he had learned from the Pythagoreans either through personal contact or through books, conceived this medical code in conformity with Pythagorean ideals.[19]

One last question remains: what is the purpose of the Oath? Is this document an ideal program with no direct bearing on reality? Or was the Oath actually administered?[20] In my opinion one need not doubt that this vow was made by many an ancient physician, that it was sworn to and regarded by them as their "Golden Rule" of conduct. If it is true that Epaminondas considered his teacher his adopted father, a physician could honor his master in the same way. If it is true that Epaminondas, the great statesman, in his life strove to practice Pythagorean virtue, a physician could do so as well.[21]

To be sure, no special societies of Pythagorean physicians are attested, no guilds are known for which Pythagorean philosophy was the statute of organization. But the covenant is a private agreement between pupil and teacher.[22] The Oath as a whole is hardly an obligation enforced upon the physician by any authority but rather one which he accepted of his own free will. It is not a legal engagement; as the wording indicates, it is a solemn promise given and vouchsafed only by the conscience of him who swears.[23] This again is in keeping with Pythagorean ethics. For the school insisted that all instruction must be based on the willingness of teacher and pupil, on voluntary

[19] That the covenant is probably modelled according to a general pattern of Pythagorean training has been suggested above, p. 49, n. 1. Nevertheless the work as a whole could be that of a physician, and the rules concerning medical conduct could hardly have been drawn by anybody except a practitioner.

[20] Cf. Jones, *op. cit.*, p. 57: "We must clearly understand, however, that the extant evidence does not prove conclusively that the *Oath* was ever actually administered. It is conceivable that it was a mere ideal, a counsel of perfection expressed in the form of an oath . . . ." Cf. also Deichgräber, *op. cit.*, p. 32 (before he uses the *Oath* as the basis for his reconstruction of the early history of Greek crafts!): "Für die sichere Beantwortung dieser Fragen (*sc.* when and where the Oath was sworn) fehlt es an näheren Nachrichten und übertragbaren Analogien."

[21] For the exemplary character of Epaminondas' life, cf. *e. g.* Nepos, *Epaminondas*, ch. 3.

[22] Cf. above, p. 40.

[23] Hirzel, *op. cit.*, p. 140, has shown that those oaths which in the end ask for reward or punishment (cf. above, p. 51) are indicative of a transition from the legal to the merely ethical sphere.

rule as well as on voluntary obedience.[24] And was not the whole reform which Pythagoras instituted a reform of the life of the individual, an appeal to man, not as a citizen, but as a private person, to lead a better, a purer, a holier existence? As Plato saw it, the Pythagorean "way of life" meant not a political or a group movement; Pythagoras wanted to stir up the conscience of the individual.[25] Throughout antiquity many responded to this summons. Certainly, in its application to the task of the physician it also found its devotees.

[24] Cf. p. 470, 35 [Diels-Kranz] (Aristoxenus) : . . . καὶ τὰς μαθήσεις τὰς ὀρθῶς γινομένας ἑκουσίως δεῖν ἔφασαν γίνεσθαι, ἀμφοτέρων βουλομένων, τοῦ τε διδάσκοντος καὶ τοῦ μανθάνοντος· ἀντιτείνοντος γὰρ ὁποτέρου δήποτε τῶν εἰρημένων οὐκ ἂν ἐπιτελεσθῆναι κατὰ τρόπον τὸ προκείμενον ἔργον.

[25] Cf. Plato, *Republic*, X, 600 a ff.; Burckhardt, *Griechische Kulturgeschichte*, III, p. 320; *Vorträge*, pp. 199 ff. It is Burckhardt who has brought out this essential point, proving it from the fact that Plato contrasted Pythagoras and Orpheus with men like Charondas and Solon. In accepting Burkhardt's characterization of the intent of Pythagorean philosophy, I do not wish to pass judgment on the controversy whether the Pythagorean movement in Italy actually was a political movement or not, cf. v. Fritz, *op. cit., passim*. Within the limits of this investigation it is not the early Pythagorean school, but Pythagoreanism as represented in the 4th century B. C. that has to be considered, cf. above, p. 18, and for this form of the Pythagorean dogma Burckhardt's interpretation is undoubtedly correct and in agreement also with the reports of Aristoxenus. Cf. also J. Burnet, *Early Greek Philosophy*⁴, 1930, p. 89 (cf. also E. Frank's review of v. Fritz' book, *American Journal of Philology*, LXIV, 1943, pp. 220 ff., which appeared when this study was already in print).

V

Conclusion

The so-called Hippocratic Oath has always been regarded as a message of timeless validity From the interpretation given it follows that the document originated in a group representing a small segment of Greek opinion. That the Oath at first was not accepted by all ancient physicians is certain. Medical writings, from the time of Hippocrates down to that of Galen, give evidence of the violation of almost every one of its injunctions. This is true not only in regard to the general rules concerning helpfulness, continence and secrecy. Such deviations one would naturally expect. But for centuries ancient physicians, in opposition to the demands made in the Oath, put poison in the hands of those among their patients who intended to commit suicide; they administered abortive remedies; they practiced surgery.

At the end of antiquity a decided change took place. Medical practice began to conform to that state of affairs which the Oath had envisaged. Surgery was separated from general practice. Resistance against suicide, against abortion, became common. Now the Oath began to be popular. It circulated in various forms adapted to the varying circumstances and purposes of the centuries.[1] Generally considered the work of the great Hippocrates, its study became part of the medical curriculum. The commentators supposed that the master had written the Oath as the first of all his books and made it incumbent on the beginner to read this treatise first.[2]

Small wonder! A new religion arose that changed the very foundations of ancient civilization. Yet, Pythagoreanism seemed to bridge the gulf between heathendom and the new belief. Christianity found

---

[1] For the manuscript tradition in general, cf. Jones, *op. cit.*, pp. 2 ff.; 12 ff.; cf. also J. H. Oliver–P. Maas, *Bulletin of the History of Medicine*, VII, 1939, pp. 315 ff. (a medical Paean); and for the *Oath* in non-medical ancient literature, cf. E. Nachmanson, *Symbolae Philologicae, O. A. Danielsson dedicatae*, Upsala, 1932, pp. 185 ff.

[2] Cf. Ps. Oribasius, *Commentarius in Aphorismos Hippocratis*, Basileae, 1535, p. 7. I need not deal here with the historical process by which ancient medical works came to be ascribed to Hippocrates, cf. L. Edelstein, The Genuine Works of Hippocrates, *Bulletin of the History of Medicine*, VII, 1939, pp. 236 ff.; cf. the same, *Problemata*, IV, ch. IV.

itself in agreement with the principles of Pythagorean ethics, its concepts of holiness and purity, justice and forbearance.[3] The Pythagorean god who forbade suicide to men, his creatures, was also the God of the Jews and the Christians. As early as in the " Teaching of the Twelve Apostles " the command was given : " Thou shalt not use philtres; thou shalt not procure abortion; nor commit infanticide." Even the Church Fathers abounded in praise of the high-mindedness of Hippocrates and his regulations for the practice of medicine.[4]

As time went on, the Hippocratic Oath became the nucleus of all medical ethics. In all countries, in all epochs in which monotheism, in its purely religious or in its more secularized form, was the accepted creed, the Hippocratic Oath was applauded as the embodiment of truth. Not only Jews and Christians, but the Arabs, the mediaeval doctors, men of the Renaissance, scientists of the Enlightenment, and scholars of the 19th century embraced the ideals of the Oath.[5] I am not qualified to outline the successive stages of this historical process. But I venture to suggest that he who undertakes to study this development will find it better understandable if he realizes that the Hippocratic Oath is a Pythagorean manifesto and not the expression of an absolute standard of medical conduct.

[3] Cf. above, p. 17, n. 40; p. 54, n. 22, where the coincidence of certain Pythagorean doctrines with Jewish (Essenian) and Christian teachings was noted. Cf. also the material collected by Meibom, op. cit., pp. 131 ff., who speaks of " Hippocratis religiositas."

[4] Cf. the so-called Διαδοχὴ τῶν δώδεκα 'Αποστόλων, The Apostolic Fathers, with an English translation by Kirsopp Lake, I, 1925, pp. 310-312 [Loeb] ; cf. also Gregory of Nazianzus, XXXV, col. 767 A [Migne] ; Hieronymus, Epist., 52, 15 (XXII, col. 539 [Migne]).

[5] It would be difficult here to substantiate this general statement; a few references to the pertinent literature must suffice. For the Jews and Arabs, cf. H. Friedenwald-G. Sarton, with reference to M. Meyerhof, Isis, XXII, 1934, pp. 222-23; cf. also Jones, op. cit., pp. 29 ff.; Deichgräber, op. cit., pp. 38 f. Some mediaeval references are collected ibid., pp. 39-40, cf. also E. Hirschfeld, Deontologische Texte des frühen Mittelalters, Archiv f. Geschichte d. Medizin, XX, 1928, p. 369. For the Renaissance and later centuries the commentaries on the Oath quoted above, p. 25, n. 72, furnish some evidence of the importance of the document; cf. besides S. V. Larkey, The Hippocratic Oath in Elizabethan England, Bulletin of the History of Medicine, IV, 1936, pp. 201 ff. Cf. also Erasmus, Methodus ad Veram Theologiam, ed. H. Holborn, 1933, p. 151; p. 180. For the 18th century, cf. e. g. J. P. Frank, The People's Misery: Mother of Diseases, H. E. Sigerist, Bulletin of the History of Medicine, IX, 1941, p. 100. Goethe, too, took over the principles of the Oath in his Wilhelm Meister, cf. Hoffmann, op. cit., pp. 18 ff.

APPENDIX
The Hippocratic Patient and His Physician
By
Herbert Newell Couch

The Hippocratean Patient and His Physician*

HERBERT NEWELL COUCH

In this essay a study is made of the attitude of the patient toward his
physician in the time of Hippocrates. His credulity is observed, his
inclination to patronize the charlatan, his recalcitrance in undergoing
treatment, as well as his more coöperative attitude in other instances.
The consistently high ideals shown by the best physicians of the Hippocratean age is also seen. Attention is called to the fact that two social
classes of patients seem to be involved, a group of substantial economic
position, for whom the writings of the theory of medicine are composed,
and a lower social class, who are identified usually by name or town in the
case histories.

In the age of Hippocrates and his immediate successors,
before medicine had degenerated into a banausic trade,
manned by slaves and reduced to a written code, there is
almost no direct evidence on which to reconstruct a picture of
Greek medical ethics. The dignity of the reputable physician,
the intellectual honesty of philosopher and scientist whose
points of view the physician combined, were in general during
the fifth and early fourth centuries deemed an adequate
safeguard for the maintenance of medical etiquette, which the
Greeks called εὐσχημοσύνη, or "good form." [1]

The task of picturing the Hippocratic patient, however, is
fraught with even greater difficulties, for there is a still more
pronounced dearth of direct testimony on the social conditions
and the point of view of the patients with whom the ancient

* I wish to acknowledge the valuable assistance of my brother, Dr. John
Harold Couch, of the Toronto General Hospital, in the preparation of this paper.

[1] W. H. S. Jones, *Hippocrates*, Loeb Class. Lib. (New York, Putnam, Vol. II,
1923), Introductory Essays v, "Ancient Medical Etiquette," xxxiii, and note 1;
see also his article, "Greek Medical Etiquette," *Proc. of the Royal Society of
Medicine*, Section of the History of Medicine, XVI (1923), 11–17. In the
Hippocratic Corpus the *Oath*, *Law*, *Physician*, *Decorum*, and *Precepts* are the
most useful treatises from which to glean information on the conduct of the
physician. The references in this article have been based on the arrangement
of the Loeb Classical Library where the material is included in it.

Greek physician came in contact. Aided, however, by a knowledge of human nature and of the domestic and civic life of the Greeks, we may perhaps be justified in extracting some significant information from the incidental references to the patients which occur in the various books of the *Corpus Hippocraticum.*

While it is true that the reputable physician was a man of honor, it must not be supposed that the age of Hippocrates was free from the malpractice of quacks and charlatans. Without anything in the nature of a licensing board it is not surprising that men in the lower ranks of medicine indulged in ques⁺'ɔnable practices, and indeed it is not always easy to draw a distinction between deliberate charlatanism and honest ignorance. In the attitude of mind of the physician of the best type, however, toward the obligations of his profession there was no compromise with dishonesty. The precepts of the leaders of the profession are normally couched in terms of the reasonable expectations of the patients themselves, for in the relation of patient and physician, as in the case of citizen and statesman, in ancient Greece the force of public opinion was enormous.

First of all we notice in the works of the ancient medical authors a continuous criticism of laxity within the profession itself, which may alienate the patient and draw censure on the art of medicine. There are in life all too many physicians who are like incompetent pilots. They are able to treat minor ailments without exposing their ignorance to laymen, but, just as in a storm the pilot destroys his ship through his own blundering ignorance, so in a severe illness the mistakes and folly of the ill trained physician become clear to all and punishment follows swiftly.[2] In medicine unsupported opinion brings in its wake censure on those who practise and destruction on those who are treated.[3] Quacks are always loath to summon their colleagues in conference when a serious

[2] *Ancient Medicine* 9 *fin.*

[3] *Decorum* 4 *med.*

situation arises,[4] but in order to safeguard the reputation of
the profession and to guard against the criticism of patients,
the practitioner who is in doubt about a case is urged to call
in a consultant.[5] Perhaps for similar reasons students in
modern medical schools are advised always to anticipate the
request of their patients for a consultation.

So definitely is the physician influenced by the attitude of
his patients that he is urged to consult laymen freely on medical
problems when his therapy may be improved thereby.[6] While
the doctor is advised to leave one of his own pupils in charge
of a case,[7] it is clear that in the absence of any regular nursing
the inmates of the house must have cared for the sick, and not
infrequently have been distinctly proficient in their duties.[8]

Especial care must be taken to avoid ridicule from fellow
practitioners or from the ever critical public. For instance,
if a patient is weak through want of nourishment and the
attending physician fails to realize it, he runs the danger of
having another physician or even a layman recognize the
condition, give food in violation of his orders, and with the
recovery of the patient of being made a laughing-stock before
all. The public, warns the medical writer, is very prone to
regard with contempt such mistakes of the physician, and they
will look upon the doctor or the layman who corrects the
original error as one who has raised the patient from the dead.[9]
So too if a physician accepts an improper case, by which is
meant a hopeless case, he will be praised by pseudo-physicians
but condemned by those who are truly scientific. The public
are apt to criticize the doctor for his attitude toward desperate

---

[4] *Precepts* 7 *med.*

[5] *Ib.* 8 *fin.* Specific advice on the dignified deportment expected from
different physicians who meet in consultation is given.

[6] *Ib.* 2 *med.*

[7] *Decorum* 17 *init.*

[8] A layman by careful questioning might even diagnose a disease. Cf.
Regimen in Acute Diseases 1 *init.* There are in the Hippocratic Corpus three
works which may be confused, viz. *Regimen* in four books, *Regimen in Acute
Diseases* in one book, and *Regimen in Health* in one book.

[9] *Regimen in Acute Diseases* 44 *fin.*

cases. This censure, says the ancient writer, is indefensible, for the public have no right to expect medicine to cope with that which is beyond its power.[10]

We must, however, deal somewhat further with the patient and the charlatan. Study and knowledge the patient has a right to demand in his doctor, for carelessness and plausible conjecture will lead to a disastrous condition, which would be harmless enough if bad doctors received their just deserts, but which unfortunately involve the innocent patients in additional suffering because of the inexperience of the doctor who has presumed to treat them.[11] The writer of the *Law* would have the state exercise authority over those who practise, since dishonor is a punishment which is little likely to deter those who have already embraced dishonorable methods.[12] The lack of agreement among physicians regarding proper treatment has also played its part in discrediting the art of medicine. Laymen have in disgust come to compare disputing physicians to rival schools of diviners, one of whom pronounces the omen of a bird seen on the right a happy one, while the other maintains the opposite.[13]   It is unfair that the physicians by their folly should themselves call upon their art such unwarranted criticism.

There are many ignorant physicians whose very ignorance is a profit to them, for they are able to persuade their neighbors of their skill and grow rich on their credulity.[14]   More serious than this, however, is the deliberate deception practised by certain quacks. The sacred disease, for instance, was first said to be supernatural by men like the magicians, purifiers, charlatans, and quacks who infested the ancient medical scene, men who claimed some superior religious knowledge pertaining to disease. They taught that the disease was

[10] *The Art* 8 *med.*

[11] *Precepts* 1 *fin.*

[12] *Law* 1 *init.*

[13] *Regimen in Acute Diseases* 8 *fin.* This matter is elaborated in some detail, with reference also to the examination of entrails.

[14] *Joints* 46 *med.*

sacred so that they might not be obliged to display their own
ignorance, and by way of treatment, in addition to idle
incantations, they added a list of silly prohibitions of foods,
drinks, and activities.[15] It is such men as these who profess
the power to call down the moon, eclipse the sun, and control
the land, the sea, and the elements. For each type of ailment
some god is accounted responsible. If the patient imitates a
goat, roars, and suffers convulsions on the right side, they
claim that the Mother of the Gods is the cause. Such follies
do they declare,[16] and such deception do they practise.

Men of questionable repute will adopt varieties of treatment
which are frowned on by the conscientious, when they can
thereby make a sensational public display. The hump-back
which is due to a fall can rarely be straightened, but incompetent and publicity-loving surgeons adopt the method of
violent shakings on a ladder, chiefly so that the mob of spec-
tators may gape at the festival and praise the performance,
without a thought for the results of the operation.[17] Not only
are such surgeons reproached, but a note of contempt for the
vulgar public creeps in here. Laymen fail constantly to
distinguish excellence in the physician, they become advocates
of novel remedies, they show stupidity in the treatment of
their own diseases, and it is really they who are responsible for
quacks attaining the name of physician.[18] Patients in their
misery are still concerned only with business. They wish to
be well so that they may return to their financial interests or
to the management of their farms. Thus they neglect their
health and swarm to the quack because of his sensational
methods, though reputable physicians are at hand.[19]

The Hippocratic patient himself presents some peculiar
problems to the physician. One of these is the force of public
opinion, with which the scientific physician is compelled at

[15] *Sacred Disease* 2 *init.*
[16] *Ib.* 3 f.
[17] *Joints* 42 *init.*
[18] *Regimen in Acute Diseases* 6.
[19] *Precepts* 7 *fin.*

times to temporize to an alarming degree. One writer tells
how he got into disrepute with his colleagues and with the
public by maintaining his opinion in a deceptive appearance
of dislocation;[20] at another time a physician counsels the
reduction of a bone which projects through the skin, a very
unsound practice involving the danger of tetanus infection,
only because the ignorant public will censure the surgeon if he
fails to make the obvious correction, and again a writer who
disapproves of hollow splints nevertheless advises their use
because the commonalty have great faith in them.[21]   Furthermore, if we remember that medical science in the time of
Hippocrates had not attained the respect that it now enjoys,
we shall understand that one of the major problems of the
ancient physician was to persuade his patients to submit to the
proper treatment.   The absence of anaesthetics and pallia-
tives, added to the natural argumentativeness of the Greek
even when ill, increased the burden of the physician,[22] in a way
little known at present except for occasional outbursts of the
anti-vaccinationists.   It is for this reason that the Hippocratic
physician emphasizes prognosis so much more than diagnosis,
for if the physician can without the aid of the patient tell with
consistent accuracy the past and present of the disease and
forecast the issue, he is likely to win the confidence of the
public.[23]   When a physician travelled from town to town
rather than establish his reputation in a given place,[24] and
when pseudo-physicians abounded, such a method of winning
quick confidence was exceedingly important.   Forecasting the

[20] *Joints* 1 *med.*

[21] *Ib.* 67 *fin; Fractures* 16 *med.*

[22] Plato frequently by way of illustration refers to the beneficial but exceedingly painful treatment by the physicians through surgery and cautery.   Cf.
Gorgias 479 a.

[23] *Prognostic* 1.

[24] The custom of travel among ancient physicians is clear from a passage in
the *Decorum* (8), where the doctor is advised to have his instruments, appliances,
knives, and bandages always ready for a call.   Particularly is he counselled to
have prepared a second and simpler physician's case, already packed in advance,
which he can take at once on a journey.

issue will do much to attain this end and it is not a difficult art to learn.[25]

Prophylactic medicine received its measure of consideration, for the ancient physician is advised to study not only the condition of the disease, but also the regimen which is beneficial to a man in health.[26] The Greek physician complained that pain alone drove his patients to consultation.[27] The obstinacy and recalcitrance of sufferers in their own treatment not infrequently tried the patience of the medical attendants. The writer of *Epidemics* says that the art of medicine deals with three factors, the disease, the patient, and the physician. The practitioner is the servant of the art, and the patient ought to coöperate with him in dealing with the ailment,[28] for a disease which arises soon after the aggravating cause, if that be known, can be most readily dealt with, providing the patient will coöperate in striking at the malady.[29] The first Aphorism of Hippocrates, "Life is short, art is long," goes on to declare that it is an obligation on the physician not only to do his own duty, but to secure the coöperation of the patient, of the attendants, and of things external.[30] While the necessity for early consultation in the incipient stages of an illness is repeatedly stressed, a full measure of coöperation was not always easy to attain, and the writer complains that patients are ready to seek treatment only when diseases have become thoroughly established.[31]

A sense of shame about certain diseases, as for instance the sacred disease, causes men, when they become conscious of an imminent attack, to run and hide from the sight of their fellows either in their own homes or in deserted places, while young children in fear of an attack run to their mothers.

[25] *Decorum* 11 *init.*
[26] *Regimen in Acute Diseases* 28–32.
[27] *Ancient Medicine* 3 *init.*
[28] *Epidemics* I, 11 *fin.*
[29] *Nature of Man* 13.
[30] *Aphorisms* I, 1.
[31] *The Art* 11 *fin.*

The non-coöperative attitude of sufferers very definitely increases the difficulty of successful treatment.[32] Inadequate hospitalization was a constant menace, particularly in cases of fractures, where the sufferers were impatient of the long period of rest required for recovery. Hence prognosis of recovery is conditional on the coöperation of the patient. Patients will be completely healed in forty days if they bring themselves to lie up for that time, if not, they will suffer more than ever.[33] Again, the patient should be well at the end of sixty days if he remains at rest;[34] or once more a warning may be added that the sufferer who will not remain quiet for forty days will recover the use of his leg only with difficulty and will be compelled to wear bandages for a long time.[35] When pain subsides patients are prone to neglect their condition, but it is the duty of the physician to warn them of the consequences.[36]

Two interesting cases reflect on the psychology of the patient toward injuries that are likely to mar his appearance. A recently broken clavicle is regarded as serious by the patient, and he hurries to his surgeon, but in time, when pain subsides and the patient finds that he is hindered neither in eating nor in working, he is apt to neglect the matter, and presently to withdraw altogether, to the frank relief of the surgeon who could not make the parts look well in any case. A broken clavicle causes a modern surgeon the same difficulty, for "if efficient, the splint is so uncomfortable that no patient will wear it, and if comfortable then it is not efficient."[37] Likewise, a broken nose alarmed the ancient sufferer since he had no wish to appear ugly, but even in such a case as this it was difficult to secure entire coöperation, for, aside from the com-

[32] *Sacred Disease* 15.
[33] *Fractures* 10 *fin.*
[34] *Ib.* 11 *fin.*
[35] *Ib.* 14 *fin.*
[36] *Joints* 9 *init.*
[37] *Ib.* 14 *init.* The quotation is from George E. Wilson, *Fractures and their Complications* (London, Macmillan, 1930), 136; cf. also 137–140.

pulsion of pain or the fear of death, men would not practice care and endurance in treatment.[38]

While we are considering the difficulties of the physician with his public, a moment's consideration should be given to another problem, namely, the deliberate and sophistic vilification of the profession which arose in certain quarters. Because some men must die under medical care the detractors of the profession assert that those who escape do so through chance and not because of the art.[39] Such sophistic arguments, which are grouped largely in the treatise on *The Art*, are answered in a similarly sophistic style. Men who make these claims, says the writer, cannot have been entirely sceptical, since they tried the art in the first place. Those who have recovered without the aid of a physician have done so because by chance they found the same remedies which a physician would have used; and, finally, if those who recover under a physician's treatment do so as the result of good luck, would it not be logical to blame ill luck rather than the physician for a fatal termination? It is more reasonable to suppose that the patient was incapable of following out the orders of the physician than that the physician erred in his instructions.[40]

In the *Decorum* the physician is counselled to be alive to the failings of his patients, who will lie to him about the regularity with which they have taken their medicine. Patients will refuse to take disagreeable things, and if they die as a result, it is never with a confession on their lips but always the blame is thrown on the doctor.[41] The patient must not be allowed to know too much of what is going on. Calmly and skilfully, cheerfully and with serenity, the physician should go about his duties, diverting the attention of his patient. Sometimes the latter must be sharply rebuked, sometimes comforted, but nothing of his future or present condition should be re-

[38] *Joints* 37 *fin.*
[39] *The Art* 4 f. and 7.
[40] *Ib.* 7.
[41] *Decorum* 14.

vealed to him.[42]   Cathartics may well be given in the gruel,
if they are such that neither taste, quantity, nor color are
likely to arouse the suspicion of the patient.[43]

That competent coöperation was occasionally forthcoming
from an intelligent patient is clear from the counsel of a writer
on surgery,[44] who says that the patient should be asked to
assist the physician with whatever part of his body is free,
and in whatever posture may be necessary to guard against
mischance in the operation.   In modern surgery a fracture
of the humerus is reduced under local rather than general
anaesthetic for the same reason, namely, so that the patient
may assi   the surgeon.   The *Regimen in Health*, that remarkable essay on prophylactic medicine, closes with the observa-
tion that the wise man will realize that his own health is his
greatest blessing, and that he himself is responsible for safe-
guarding it.[45]   In view of some of the observations already
made and of the fact that anaesthetics were little used, this
attitude toward the patient bespeaks an intelligent and co-
operative clientele of a high order.

Finally, we have some evidence of the deportment of the
physician which will be expected and demanded by his patients.   Ostentation,[46] exhibition of confusion, and indulgence in much idle talk are particularly to be condemned in
the practice of medicine.[47]   The physician is advised also that
he must not, in order to extend his clientele, wear elaborate
headdress nor use exotic perfumes.   If he indulges in extravagant novelty he will only win disrepute for himself, although
a little indulgence in these whims may fall within the limits
of good taste.   The dignity of the physician need not, however,
prevent him from trying to please his patients.[48]   The doctor

[42] *Ib.* 16.

[43] *Regimen in Acute Diseases* 23 *fin.*

[44] *In the Surgery* 3 *fin.*

[45] *Regimen in Health* 9.

[46] *Decorum* 5.

[47] *Joints* 44 *fin.*

[48] *Precepts* 10.

ought to practise a genial ready wit, for the sick and the
healthy alike find austerity or dourness repulsive, but gossip
among his patients is forbidden, for it will only draw criticism
on his art.   He should be prepared in advance for his conduct
in the sick-room, where the patient will observe the manner in
which the doctor sits, the mode of his dress, his concise brief
speech, his bedside manner, his attentiveness undiverted by
irrelevancies, his ability to deal with objections and to repri-
mand disturbances, the measure of his self-control, and his
readiness to do all that is necessary.[49]   Unremitting attention
to the critical disposition of the patient is earnestly urged on
the doctor.   From the treatise on the *Physician* we find similar
counsel advocated for psychological reasons.   He is again
urged to practise the virtues of cleanliness, neatness, prudence,
and kindness, to avoid undue forwardness, harshness, and
vulgarity.   He must remember that the relationship of patient
and physician is a very intimate one, and that women and
maidens very precious in the sight of others will come to him
for advice.   His conduct must, therefore, be at all times in
keeping with the dignity of a gentleman.   Lastly, since the
public will expect the physician to heal himself if he is to heal
others, the medical man ought to contrive to look healthy and
to be as plump as nature intended that he should be.[50]   From
the *Oath* we gather the well-known pledge that the physician
will enter each house only to aid the suffering, that he will
refrain from all intentional misconduct and from all gossip.
The *Decorum* [51] ends with a summary of the conduct in wisdom,
in medicine, and in the arts in general, which will make for
reputation and honor.   To the practice of these the physician
is commended.

Another and rather different phase of this study remains.
It is an examination of the social condition, particularly as to
social distinction, of the patients to whom reference is made

[49] *Decorum* 12.
[50] *Physician* 1.
[51] *Decorum* 18.

in the Hippocratic Corpus, and it is based, firstly, upon the incidental references to the circumstances of an illness, or to the equipment used in the treatment of a disease, and secondly, upon particular men and women who are mentioned by name or otherwise definitely identified as illustrating a certain condition or a type of disease.

It is clear that the good physician of Hippocrates' time was not only a man of science but in the community he was a person of some social distinction. He was meticulous in the maintenance of medical proprieties. Advertising was forbidden, although it was permissible for a physician to grant free medical service to a town, and in turn this was likely to lead to civic recognition and handsome emolument.[52] The career of Democedes of Croton will serve as an illustration of the repute that a skilled physician enjoyed in various cities.[53] The physician was conscious of the dignity of his profession. Wisdom and medicine, says the writer of *Decorum*,[54] should go hand in hand, for the physician who dedicates himself to wisdom is like to a god. To this conception should be added the fact that ancient medical etiquette, according to the general treatises, emphasized the welfare of the patient even more than the maintenance of the dignity of the profession.[55]

A moment's reflection on the normal state of privation which existed in ancient Greek society will make it possible to evaluate more justly the few references that can be gathered on the material and social conditions of the Hippocratean patient. "Poverty," says Herodotus (vii, 102), "has ever been the sister of Greece." Zimmern,[56] deprecating the tendency to regard the Greeks as the pioneers of civilization and therefore blessed with all the comforts of modern life, gives a startling picture of the truly primitive, and to modern sensibilities, appalling state of want in which the Greeks lived:

[52] See W. H. S. Jones, *op. cit.* ii, xxxiv, note 2 (see *supra*, note 1).

[53] Herodotus iii, 125–135.

[54] *Decorum* 5.

[55] See W. H. S. Jones, *op. cit.* ii, xxxv (*supra*, note 1).

[56] A. E. Zimmern, *The Greek Commonwealth*[4] (Oxford, Clarendon, 1924), 215.

"It is easy enough to think away railways and telegraphs and gas works and tea and advertisements and bananas. But we must peel off more than this. We must imagine houses without drains, beds without sheets or springs, rooms as cold, or as hot, as the open air, only draughtier, meals that began and ended with pudding. . . . We must learn to tell time without watches, to cross rivers without bridges, and seas without a compass, to fasten our clothes (or rather our two pieces of cloth) with two pins instead of rows of buttons, to wear our shoes or sandals without stockings, to warm ourselves over a pot of ashes, to judge open-air plays or law-suits on a cold winter's morning, to study poetry without books, geography without maps, and politics without newspapers. In a word we must learn how to be civilized without being comfortable."

Ill equipped the Greek may have been, but he was not necessarily unhappy, and the above extract has been quoted simply to show his attitude toward physical comfort, so that as material conveniences are mentioned in connection with the treatment of the sick they may be understood in relation to Greek life and not to modern standards. One observes then a solicitude on the part of the Greek medical writer for his patients, and an ability on the part of the public themselves to supply material comforts in illness, which suggest that the patients for whom the theory of medicine is composed belonged to the more prosperous classes of ancient society.

The patients are not infrequently those who patronized the palaestra and the gymnasium. In fact the physician who has come to a new town is advised to acquaint himself at once with the manner of life of his prospective patients, whether they are given to heavy drinking and accustomed to take more than one full meal a day (in itself an indication of high living) and are therefore sluggish, or whether they are fond of athletics, vigorous, given to hearty eating and restrained drinking.[57] In the First Constitution of the *Epidemics* [58] it is stated that

[57] *Airs, Waters, Places* 1 *fin.*
[58] *Epidemics* I, 1 *fin.*

the victims of the pestilence were chiefly youths and young
men in their prime, especially those who frequented the
wrestling schools and gymnasia. The preservation of good
health among athletes [59] is cited as one of the duties of the
physician, although in the *Aphorisms* [60] a warning against
too high a pitch of bodily perfection is sounded, since any
change must necessarily be for the worse. Moderate exercise,
including wrestling and running on the circular or double track,
is advised in certain cases; [61] athletes should vary their training
in accordance with the seasons; [62] the desirability of observing
a patient as he strips and performs his exercises so that the
physician may wisely prescribe for him is once mentioned; [63]
athletes are cited as a class who because of greater "innate"
heat require more food; [64] a man who has been habituated to
the palaestra is suggested as a suitable person to perform an
operation on the spine; [65] and finally, in the discussion of the
posture to be used in treating fractures the illustration adopted
is that of athletics.[66] These illustrations have been grouped
and cited without elaboration simply as evidence of the substantial social stratum of the patients who are busied about
the normal Greek life of the palaestra and the gymnasium.

A number of scattered and fortuitous references show the
solicitude of the physician for the physical and mental comfort
of his patients.[67] While some patients will ask for unreasonable attentions, the physician should not rebuke them too
severely.[68] The physician should take the lead in dispelling

[59] *Regimen in Acute Diseases* 9.

[60] *Aphorisms* I, 3.

[61] *Regimen* I, 35 *med.*

[62] *Regimen in Health* 7 *init.*

[63] *Regimen* I, 2 *med.*

[64] *Aphorisms* I, 15.

[65] *Joints* 47 *med.*

[66] *Fractures* 2 *med.* The reference is to the different natural postures assumed
in various athletic contests.

[67] *Precepts* 3-13 contains considerable information on the relation of patient
and physician.

[68] *Precepts* 5.

the despondency of his patients who, when they are ill, are apt to become depressed and give up the struggle for life.[69] The physician must exercise the greatest tact and consideration for the financial condition of his patients in the matter of fees. A stranger in distress should be treated for the love of the art and for the satisfaction of conferring a benefit even though no remuneration can be expected.[70] A patient should not be distressed by discussing fees with him before treatment, lest an acute condition be aggravated by worry. The ancient writer apparently does not consider the possibility that the arrangement in advance of an equable fee with a reasonable physician might mitigate worry over the financial aspect of the illness. That the Greek physician occasionally met difficulty and ingratitude in attempting to collect his accounts is to be inferred from the admonition that it is better to reproach patients who have been saved than to extort money from those who are critically ill. Seek not profit but reputation.[71] No patient should be disturbed during or immediately after a crisis nor should experiments be tried on him,[72] and a patient who is on a starvation diet ought not to be fatigued.[73] Two references to the careful use of surgical apparatus to avoid irritation to the patient may be added. The first arises in considering the use of hollow splints, which the writer considers of dubious value and of considerable discomfort to the patient unless something soft is inserted between the wood and the limb.[74] Secondly, in the matter of a broken jaw a piece of Carthaginian leather is cut and attached to the jaw with gum, since it is more agreeable to the patient than glue.[75] The intricacies of bandaging need not be related. For the moment a question of greater interest is the aesthetic feeling of the

[69] *Ib.* 9 *med.*
[70] *Ib.* 6.
[71] *Ib.* 4.
[72] *Aphorisms* I, 20.
[73] *Ib.* II, 16.
[74] *Fractures* 16 *med.*
[75] *Joints* 33 *init.*

patient who prefers gum to glue on his jaw, and the consideration of the physician in prescribing it.

There should be included a brief summary of some apparatus that is used, or treatment that is advised, which presumes some capacity on the part of the patient to follow the not inexpensive course of treatment.[76] Change of climate, place, and mode of life are suggested for the treatment of epilepsy in the young.[77] In the *Regimen in Health* [78] there is detailed advice on food and customs, which presumes the ability of the patient to carry out the instructions. Vapor baths, or even aromatic vapor baths, something which would not ┝ ˙ easy to obtain in the most meagre circumstances, are prescribed again and again for a variety of ailments.[79] Elsewhere the use of the bath is discussed at length,[80] and it is conceded that few homes have suitable apparatus or proper attendants for the bath, so that its use will necessarily be restricted to the more affluent. An improperly conducted bath may do no little harm. The necessary equipment embraces a covered place in which no smoke is found, and plenty of hot water. If soap is used it should be warm and much greater in quantity than usual. Furthermore, the distance to the basin should be short, and the basin easy to enter and to leave. The bather should remain at rest himself and leave all pouring of water and rubbing to the attendants. Sponges rather than a scraper should be used and the body should be anointed before it is quite dry.[81] The habits of the patient himself should be considered, for the use of the bath without proper facilities is likely to do more harm than good.[82] Simple hot baths are recommended, sometimes of themselves,

[76] The ancient surgeon had, of course, considerable equipment himself. See *Fractures*, and *Joints, passim*.

[77] *Aphorisms* II, 45.

[78] Especially chaps. 2–5.

[79] *Regimen* I, 35 *med;* III, 72; IV, 89 *med; Aphorisms* v, 28; *Joints* 47 *init.*

[80] *Regimen in Acute Diseases* 65–68.

[81] *Ib.* 65 *init.*

[82] *Ib.* 67 *f.*

sometimes as a substitute if vapor baths prove impracticable,[83] while at times anointing with oil and sleep on a soft bed is prescribed in conjunction with the bath.[84] The value of different types of bath, whether fresh water or salt, hot or cold, is once discussed in some detail.[85] One physician can see value in occasional indulgence in moderate drunkenness and other vices in addition to warm baths and a soft bed together with a diminution of exercise to effect relaxation.[86] The bed comes in for a good deal of attention. Sometimes a soft one is recommended,[87] and again it should be hard.[88]

It is the duty of the physician to consider the nature of the bed, the season of the year, the needs of the patient, which may demand that he be put in a place open to the breezes or in a covered place beneath the ground. Noises and smells, particularly that of wine,[89] are injurious and should be avoided. Perhaps the classic example of luxurious treatment occurs in the *Regimen*,[90] where with great detail the procedure is described, a moderately warm bath, a drink of soft wine, an ample, well planned dinner, a second drink of well diluted soft wine, a short stroll, and finally sleep on a soft bed. It is suggested in the light of these examples which have been quoted, and with a mind on the normal poverty of material resources in a Greek home, that the more or less elaborate treatment prescribed in this theory of medicine presumes a clientele drawn at least from the more prosperous social classes. That, of course, does not necessarily mean the aristocracy. In fact we have two references in which the patients are rather definitely identified as belonging to the class of skilled artisans. A man whose shoulder has been broken will, for instance, on recovery be able to operate a bow-drill, a saw, a pick, or a

[83] *Regimen* II, 66 *med;* III, 72 *med;* 76 *med;* 81 *med;* 83 *fin.*
[84] *Regimen* III, 80 *fin;* 83.
[85] *Ib.* II, 57 *init.*
[86] *Ib.* III, 85 *init.*
[87] *Ib.* IV, 89 *med;* 90 *fin.*
[88] *Ib.* III, 68 *med.*   Bed-clothing is mentioned in *Prognostic* 4.
[89] *Decorum* 15.
[90] *Regimen* II, 66.

spade, none of which demand much lifting of the elbow.[91] Less specific but similar is the inference to be drawn from the passage in the *Nature of Man*,[92] where in certain conditions appearing in men over thirty-five years of age it is suggested that in their youth they must have been hard-working, industrious, and vigorous, but that afterwards when they have given up their strenuous toil their flesh has become soft and weak.

The physician should learn the proper method of treating those who suffer from frequent dislocation of the shoulder, for many have on this account been debarred from the athletic contests, or rendered useless for war, though otherwise well fitted for both activities.[93] For the treatment of dislocation various methods of manual manipulation are recommended, which will be particularly useful at the palaestra, since no additional apparatus need be furnished.[94]

The well stuffed leather pillow which will yield only slightly when a patient rests his head on it while his dislocated jaw is set;[95] the leather or linen pillows which are placed across the ladder on which the humpback is treated;[96] the gold wire which is recommended for fastening together dislodged or loosened teeth;[97] the remarkable chapter on the treatment of club foot, with its detailed instructions on the types of footwear which should be successively used,[98] all argue a comparative degree of economic prosperity among the patients for whom they are prescribed.

A final group of patients has purposely been isolated to this point, namely, those who are mentioned by name or individually identified in connection with the discussion of diseases,

[91] *Joints* 12 *fin*.

[92] *Nature of Man* 12 *init*.

[93] *Joints* 11 *init*.

[94] *Ib*. 4 *med*. For instance, if the patient is too light to make a counterweight of his own body, a boy may cling to him from behind.

[95] *Ib*. 30 *fin*.

[96] *Ib*. 43 *med*.

[97] *Ib*. 32 *med*.

[98] *Ib*. 62 *fin*.

and who are found in greatest number in the lists of case histories in the *Epidemics*. No attempt is made in this paper to diagnose the diseases for two reasons, firstly, because in any case no self-respecting modern physician will content himself with the casual or even careful diagnosis which a colleague makes of any disputed ancient Greek disease, and secondly, because such a study is unlikely to yield anything of value about the social condition of the Hippocratean patient and his relationship with his physician, for such diseases as gout and chlorosis, which might afford some evidence of the mode of life of a class, seem not to have occurred to any great extent. Where significant circumstances in any given case are recorded they are mentioned in their proper relationship.

An ordered classification of the patients who are named or otherwise identified should first be attempted. Some sixty-five of these have been assembled, with one exception, from the *Epidemics* and the case histories included therein. Of these fully fifty per cent are not even named, but are perfunctorily identified by reference to the person with whom they lodged or to the place where they lay sick. The list, however, may be analyzed still more systematically. Seven men are named,[99] but about these nothing further is told except that one, Myllus, is coupled with the slave of Erato, and another, Xenophanes, presumably kept lodgers.[100] In addition to this first group three more men are themselves named and are further identified by the name of their fathers.[101] Five women or girls, who are not themselves mentioned by name, are identified by the names of their fathers,[102] and five other women, themselves nameless, are identified by the names of their hus-

---

[99] Viz. Myllus (*Epidemics* I, 15); Xenophanes (*ib.* 17); Critias (*ib.*); Epaminondas (*ib.* 21); Silenus (*ib.*); Herophon (*Epidemics* I, *case* 3); Meton (*ib. case* 7).

[100] *Ib.* 17.

[101] Viz. Antiphon the son of Critobulus (*ib.* 15); Euagon the son of Daitharses (*ib.* 20); Philiscus the son of Antagoras (*ib.* 21).

[102] Viz. the daughters of Telebulus (*ib.* 16), Daitharses (*ib.*), Philo (*ib.* 19), Aglaidas (*ib.* 20), Euyanax (*Epidemics* III, *case* 6).

bands.[103] These twenty persons it will be best to dismiss without comment. In no case is anything of marked significance told about their social condition, and where only a name is given, whether it be that of the patient, the father, or the husband, there is no basis on which to draw any conclusions at all about the position of the patient in his city.

From the remaining forty-five cases, however, some information can be extracted. Four men are identified as lying ill at the home of another, whether landlord or friend cannot be determined.[104] Three of these are named. Bion lay sick at the home of Silenus;[105] Phanocritus at the home of Gnathon the fuller;[106] Chaerion at the home of Demaenetus;[107] and, finally, an unidentified woman suffering from angina lay sick in the home of Aristion.[108] From this list it is clear that the patients were at least unimportant enough to be identified by the names of the men in whose homes they were found, rather than in and of themselves. One of these was a fuller. The patients were not themselves householders.

Two further cases are found where the patients are known to have been lodgers. Cratis lived in that capacity with Xenophanes,[109] and an unnamed woman lodged with Tisamenus.[110] Of the social condition of these patients the same arguments are applicable as those applied to the previous group. Seven patients are identified by the city in which they lived. Of these four are mentioned by name,[111] and

[103] Viz. the wives of Mnesistratus (*Epidemics* I, 17), Philinus (*ib. case* 4), Epicrates (*ib. case* 5), Dromeades (*ib. case* 11), Hicetas (*Epidemics* III, *case* 11).

[104] See E. Littré, *Hippocrates* (Paris [1839–1861] VIII, vii–xxix and x, xxix–xxxii) for a discussion of the social position of some of the patients, and a consideration of the opinions of his predecessors.

[105] *Epidemics* I, 15 and 17.

[106] *Ib.* 21.

[107] *Epidemics* III, *case* 5. There is some uncertainty about the reading of the proper name, which does not affect the argument.

[108] *Ib. case* 7.

[109] *Epidemics* I, 17.

[110] *Epidemics* III, *case* 9.

[111] Viz. Hermippus of Clazomenae (*Epidemics* I, 20); Crito of Thasos (*ib. case* 9); Pericles of Abdera (*Epidemics* III, *Sixteen Cases*, *case* 6); Heropythus of Abdera (*ib. case* 9).

the three others are more vaguely referred to as "a bald man in Larisa,"[112] "a maiden in Larisa,"[113] and "a woman in Cyzicus."[114] Perhaps in the case of these too it is unfair to draw any conclusions as to their position in the city, although it must be recognized that the identification is perfunc ory, and therefore it might be argued with some reason that the social class is not high.

Eight other cases, however, are recorded, in which not only is the city mentioned but some other information about the place of residence or the nature of the illness is known, and one is here on a little firmer ground in seeking to draw conclusions. The pertinent facts about some of these cases may be recalled. Philistes of Thasos[115] had long suffered from pains in the head, which finally had caused stupor and drove him to his bed. He had been drinking heavily and this caused continuous fever. He died on the fifth day. Nicodemus of Abdera[116] was attacked by fever after heavy drunkenness and debauchery. His fever passed with the crisis on the twenty-fourth day. An unnamed youth of Meliboea,[117] after a long period of heavy drinking and debauchery, took to his bed. Death came on the twenty-fourth day. Chaerion, who has already been mentioned,[118] likewise suffered from fever which followed heavy drinking. These cases afford evidence of acute alcoholism among a disreputable class of society.

Of another group of patients, who are identified chiefly by reference to the city in which they lived, these further fragments of information are available. An unnamed girl in Abdera[119] lay sick by the Sacred Way for twenty-seven days. Anaxion of Abdera[120] lay sick of acute fever for thirty-four

[112] *Ib. case* 5.
[113] *Ib. case* 12.
[114] *Ib. case* 14.
[115] *Epidemics* III, *case* 4.
[116] *Epidemics* III, *Sixteen Cases, case* 10.
[117] *Ib. case* 16.
[118] *Epidemics* III, *case* 5.
[119] *Epidemics* III, *Sixteen Cases, case* 7.
[120] *Ib. case* 8.

days by the Thracian Gate. In this case it is stated that on
the eighth day the physician bled him on the arm, scant but
welcome information on the extent to which the physician
cared personally for these patients. An unnamed woman of
melancholy disposition, who lived in Thasos near Pylades'
place on the plain,[121] "after a sorrow with a reason behind it,"
took to her bed, and on the first day of her illness, when there
was an intermission in her frequent convulsions, she wandered
about uttering obscenities. Apollonius of Abdera [122] apparently suffered from acute stomach trouble, for his condition
was aggravated by unwise drinking of cow's, goat's, and sheep's
milk, as well as by his regimen in general. In Thasos the
wife of Delearces,[123] who was seized with acute fever "after a
sorrow," lay sick on the plain. She seems to have suffered
from nervousness and hysteria with symptoms of athetosis,
weeping, laughing, fumbling, and picking hairs from the bed-
clothes. She had attendants.

The patients mentioned in this last group evidently had the
most meagre living accommodations, and in some instances
they apparently were quite without shelter. In fact, another
group of patients is to be identified principally by the place
where they were found ill. It will be well to cite the significant
facts for each of these also. Two brothers who suffered at the
same time lay sick near Epigenes' summer house; [124] Clea-
nactides lay sick near the temple of Heracles; [125] an unnamed
Clazomenian was attacked by fever and lay sick by the wall
of Phrynichides; [126] a woman three months pregnant, unidentified by name or city, was seized with fever and lay sick beside
the shore; [127] Melidia lay sick by the temple of Hera; [128]

[121] *Ib. case* 11.
[122] *Ib. case* 13.
[123] *Ib. case* 15.
[124] *Epidemics* I, 20.
[125] *Ib. case* 6.
[126] *Ib. case* 10.
[127] *Ib. case* 13.
[128] *Ib. case* 14.

Hermocrates lay sick with fever by the New Wall; [129] an unnamed man, who had suffered for a long time with pains in
the head, was seized with fever and lay sick in the garden of
Delearces; [130] an unnamed youth of about twenty, following
unaccustomed weariness, labor, and running, was seized with
a fever and lay sick by the Liars' Market.[131]   He died on the
seventh day.   Also by the Liars' Market a girl of about seven-
teen gave birth to a child, and lay sick there until the four-
teenth day, when she died.[132]   Three cases are reported from
Thasos.   A foreigner from Paros lay sick above the temple of
Artemis; [133] an unnamed woman on the third day after giving
birth to a child was taken with acute fever and lay by the Cold
Water,[134] where apparently she remained for nearly three
months; Pythion, after toil, weariness, and a careless mode of
life, was seized with acute fever and lay sick above the temple
of Heracles.[135]   Lastly, the wife of Epicrates gave birth to a
child near the statue of the founder of the city.[136]   The
evidence of this group, who have been cited without elaboration of the inferences, points again to the poorer and needier
sections of the population.

There may be added the names of six patients who are
differentiated from the preceding because the place of their
residence is specified, rather than simply the place of their
illness, which may be a very different thing, as in a few cases
is clearly testified.   Cratistorax lived near the temple of
Heracles,[137] Pantacles near the temple of Dionysus.[138]   One
may suspect that the social distinction between the two dis-

[129] *Epidemics* III, *case* 2.

[130] *Ib. case* 3.

[131] *Ib. case* 8.

[132] *Ib. case* 12.

[133] *Epidemics* III, *Sixteen Cases, case* 1.

[134] *Ib. case* 2.

[135] *Ib. case* 3.

[136] *Epidemics* I, *case* 5.   This may refer to the temple of the patron god of
the city.

[137] *Ib.* 21.

[138] *Ib.*

tricts was not great. Philiscus lived beside the Wall.[139] Silenus, a lad of twenty, following over-exertion, heavy drinking, and exercise at the wrong time, was seized with fever. His home was on the Square near the place of Eualcidas.[140] Erasinus lived beside Boötes Gorge,[141] and Python beside the temple of Earth.[142]

Two patients are identified only by the disease from which they suffered. One was a man who ate and drank too much when he was heated,[143] as a result of which he died on the eleventh day; the other was a patient suffering from phrenitis,[144] about whom nothing else of interest is known.

Finally, and of some significance, five slaves are mentioned among the patients. They are not themselves named, but they are identified by the persons to whom they belonged, viz. "the slave of Erato";[145] "the slave of Areton";[146] "the female servant of Scymnus the fuller";[147] "a woman of the household of Pantimedes";[148] and "the slave of Antigenes."[149] No further significant facts about them or their masters are recorded.

This much information is then available about the patients who are cited as examples of specific diseases. Aside from those who are simply named or identified by city, there are men and women who are lodgers or sojourners in the homes of others, women who give birth to children in gardens and by public roads, men who lie ill by the Liars' Market, men whose ailments have been aggravated by drunkenness and immorality, servants, and slaves. With no desire to force unduly any of

---

[139] *Ib. case* 1.
[140] *Ib. case* 2.
[141] *Ib. case* 8.
[142] *Epidemics* iii, *case* 1.
[143] *Epidemics* i, *case* 12.
[144] *Epidemics* iii, *Sixteen Cases, case* 4.
[145] *Epidemics* i, 15.
[146] *Ib.* 17.
[147] *Ib.* 21.
[148] *Epidemics* iii, *case* 10.
[149] *Humors* 20 *fin.*

the evidence that has been cited, and mindful of the comparative simplicity of Greek domestic life at all times, nevertheless
one is forced to conclude that the named patients of the Hippocratic Corpus are the poorer or charity class of the physician's
clientele.   They would correspond to the public ward patients
of a modern university hospital, who are necessarily the sub-
jects of the medical clinics.   It may be supposed also that in
the writings which deal with the practice of medicine, in which
the deference of the physician toward his public is constantly
uppermost and in which no names are mentioned, the writer
has refrained from personal mention out of regard to the wishes
and feelings of his patients.

Very little is known about the practical clinical experience
of the medical apprentice, but in this connection marked
attention should be given to the concluding chapter of the
Physician,[150] in which the prospective surgeon is strongly
advised to seek practical experience in this branch of medicine
by attaching himself to a mercenary expedition.   The advice
in itself indicates that the essay was written after 400 B.C.,
but it is of considerable importance in estimating the procedure
of the surgeon in seeking experience away from the ranks of
established practice.

It should finally be pointed out that there is no reason to
believe that the ancient physician was any less attentive or
conscientious in his treatment of the poorer classes than is his
modern colleague.   The Greek physician was essentially a
scientist, with the intellectual curiosity of all Greek men of
letters, and he was sustained both in the theory of medicine
and in its practice among all classes by an insatiable curiosity
to know the truth.

[150] *Physician* 14.

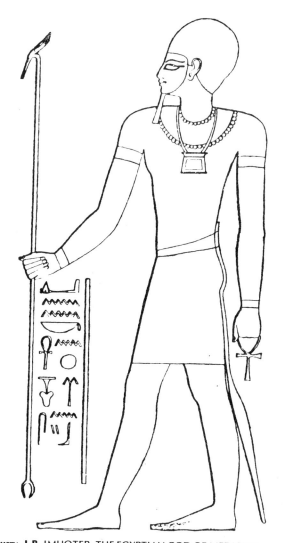

Hurry, J.B. IMHOTEP: THE EGYPTIAN GOD OF MEDICINE.
Who was Imhotep? The ancient hieroglyphic texts have preserved the
memory of a distinguished magician-physician with this name from
the reign of King Zoser (Third Dynasty) down to the Ptolemaic and
Roman periods. His records extend over a large part of the history of
ancient Egypt. The author traces the fortunes of Imhotep from the
period of his human activity through the subsequent periods when he
was looked upon first as a demigod and finally as one of the full
deities of the Egyptian pantheon. A beautiful and well-documented
story, based on ancient texts, archaeological excavations and
discoveries and monuments of Egyptian Art.

ISBN 0-89005-239-5. xvi + 120 pp. + 17 pls. $12.50

ΙΣΥΛΛΟΣΣΩΚΡΑΤΕΥΣΕΠΙΔΑΥΡΙΟΣΑΝΕΘΗΚΕ
ΑΠΟΛΛΩΝΙΜΑΛΕΑΤΑΙΚΑΙΑΣΚΛΑΠΙΩΙ
ΔΑΜΟΣΕΙΣΑΡΙΣΤΟΚΡΑΤΙΑΝΑΝΔΡΑΣΑΙΠΡΟΑΓΟΙΚΑΛΩΣ
ΑΥΤΟΣΙΣΧΥΡΟΤΕΡΟΣΟΡΘΟΥΤΑΙΓΑΡΕΞΑΝΔΡΑΓΑΘΙΑΣ
ΑΙΔΕΤΙΣΚΑΛΩΣΠΡΟΑΧΘΕΙΣΟΙΓΓΑΝΟΙΠΟΝΗΡΙΑΣ
ΠΑΛΙΝΕΠΑΓΚΡΟΥΩΝΚΟΛΑΙΩΝΔΑΜΟΣΑΣΦΑΛΕΣΤΕΡΟΣ

Gaertringen Hiller de Fr. INSCRIPTIONES EPIDAURI.
The volume contains all the inscriptions discovered in the excavations
of the famous sanctuary of Apollo and Asklepios near the ancient city
of Epidaurus. A group of Greek texts that revised our knowledge about
ancient medicine and its practices and added also some very valuable
hymns to the 'Anthologia Lyrica' (*Issyllos if Epidaurus, etc.*).
(R. 1929)
  ISBN 0-89005-207-7. xxxix + 220 pp. + 4 pls. $25.00

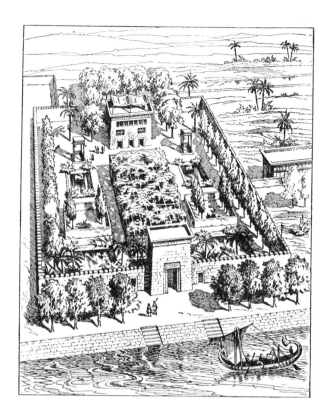

Budge E.A. Wallis. HERB-DOCTORS AND PHYSICIANS IN THE ANCIENT WORLD. The Divine Origin of the Craft of the Herbalist.

"The herb-doctors and physicians of Sumer, Babylon, Assyria and Egypt have proclaimed with no uncertain voice that their craft was founded by the gods, who taught men the curative properties of water, herbs and plants and oils, and who were themselves the first practitioners. And for the last 5000 years men in every civilized country have regarded the divine art of healing as the greatest of the gods' gifts to men." From the *Prefactory note* by E.A. Wallis Budge.

ISBN 0-89005-252-2

$10.00

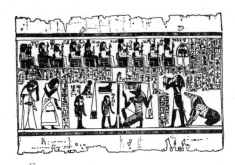

Bryan, Cyril. ANCIENT EGYPTIAN MEDICINE: THE PAPYRUS EBERS. This curious book—the oldest papyrus book in existence, it is claimed—was written by an ancient Egyptian physician. It contains the best information available on Egyptian medical practices. Though crocodile teeth and some of the other ingredients may be rather difficult to obtain, the venturesome may want to experiment with a few of the remedies suggested. (R 1930) See also J.G. Milne.

ISBN 0-89005-004-X. xxxvi + 167 pp. + 16 pl. *$12.50*

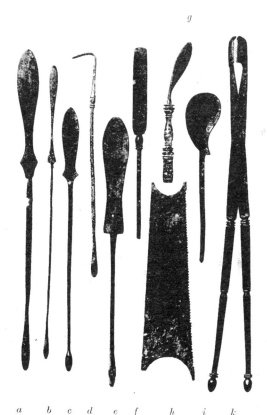

g

a   b   c   d   e   f   h   i   k

Milne, J.G. SURGICAL INSTRUMENTS IN GREEK AND ROMAN TIMES.
The best collection of information from both literary sources *and* archaeological monuments on the types of ancient surgical instruments used by the physicians of the Greco-Roman world. If there were actually a brance of archaeology that could be called "medical archaeology" or "surgical archaeology," this would be the first and fundamental book on the subject. Fifty-four plates illustrate the surgical instruments discussed in this valuable reference work. See also Cyril Bryan, *Ancient Egyptian Medicine.* (R 1907)

ISBN 0-89005-127-5. 187 pp. + 54 pl. *$20.00*